# Osseointegration: On Continuing Synergies in Surgery, Prosthodontics, and Biomaterials

# OSSEOINTEGRATION

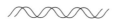

## On Continuing Synergies in
## Surgery · Prosthodontics · Biomaterials

Edited by

GEORGE A. ZARB, BChD, DDS, MS, MS, FRCD(C)

TOMAS ALBREKTSSON, MD, PhD, ODhc

GERALD BAKER, DDS, MS, FRCD(C)

STEVEN E. ECKERT, DDS, MS

CLARK STANFORD, DDS, PhD

DENNIS P. TARNOW, DDS

ANN WENNERBERG, DDS, PhD

**Quintessence Publishing Co, Inc**

Chicago, Berlin, Tokyo, London, Paris, Milan, Barcelona,
Istanbul, São Paulo, Mumbai, Moscow, Prague, and Warsaw

Library of Congress Cataloging-in-Publication Data

Osseointegration : on continuing synergies in surgery, prosthodontics, and biomaterials / edited by George A. Zarb ... [et al.].
    p. ; cm.
  Includes bibliographical references and index.
  ISBN 978-0-86715-479-5 (hardcover)
  1. Osseointegrated dental implants. 2. Osseointegration. I. Zarb, George A. (George Albert), 1938-
  [DNLM: 1. Dental Implantation, Endosseous—trends. 2. Osseointegration. 3. Dental Implants—trends. WU 640 O846 2008]
  RK667.I45O92 2008
  617.6'92—dc22
                          2008029460

© 2008 Quintessence Publishing Co, Inc

Quintessence Publishing Co Inc
4350 Chandler Drive
Hanover Park, IL 60133
www.quintpub.com

Editor: Kathryn Funk
Design: Annette McQuade
Production: Sue Robinson

Printed in China

# TABLE OF CONTENTS

# PREFACE

Per-Ingvar Brånemark introduced the concept of osseointegrated dental implants and raised the bar for management of dental and orofacial deficits. As a result, long-term clinical outcomes from the technique's scrupulously applied surgical and prosthodontic protocols ushered in a new and exciting dental treatment era, particularly for partially and completely edentulous patients.

The method's ensuing clinical virtuosity evolved from rigorous scientific documentation and critical appreciation of two very compelling considerations: first, the realization that a particular metal, commercially pure titanium, designed in different macroscopic and microscopic forms, offers the potential to become strongly rooted in bone under controlled conditions; and second, the development of specified surgical tissue management and prosthodontic loading protocols to induce and maintain the desired interfacial osteogenesis.

Subsequent routine dental use of osseointegration resulted from a long research voyage in a vessel made seaworthy by the synergistic efforts of numerous clinical scientists. The scholarly journey was a long and fruitful one since its Gothenburg inception and subsequent launch via the Toronto Conference of 1982. A number of this book's writers were crew members on that first journey, while others joined at a later time. Together we have weathered both fair and heavy conditions as we tended to—and sometimes even replaced—the vessel's planks while staying afloat.

The clinical journey continues to be an exciting one, and this monograph seeks to be a log of the important ports visited and revisited. We hope that a synthesis of these fascinating venues provides a useful guide for those readers who plan their treatment voyages to similar destinations.

# Contributors

**Tomas Albrektsson**, MD, PhD, ODhc
Professor and Head
Department of Biomaterials
University of Gothenburg
Gothenburg, Sweden

**Nikolai Attard**, BChD, MSc, PhD
Lecturer
Department of Restorative Dentistry
Faculty of Dental Surgery
University of Malta
Msida, Malta

**Gerald Baker**, DDS, MS, FRCD(C)
Head
Division of Oral and Maxillofacial Surgery
Department of Dentistry
Mount Sinai Hospital
Toronto, Ontario, Canada
Assistant Professor
Oral and Maxillofacial Surgery and
    Implant Prosthodontic Unit
Faculty of Dentistry
University of Toronto
Toronto, Ontario, Canada

**S. Ross Bryant**, DDS, MSc, PhD, FRCD(C)
Assistant Professor
Division of Prosthodontics and Dental Geriatrics
Department of Oral Health Sciences
Faculty of Dentistry
University of British Columbia
Vancouver, British Columbia, Canada

**David Chvartszaid**, DDS, MSc
Prosthodontist
Resident
Department of Periodontology
Faculty of Dentistry
University of Toronto
Toronto, Ontario, Canada

**Sang-Choon Cho**, DDS
Associate Director of Clinical Research
Assistant Clinical Professor
Department of Periodontology and Implant Dentistry
College of Dentistry
New York University
New York, New York

**Lesley David**, DDS, FRCD(C)
Staff Surgeon
Division of Oral and Maxillofacial Surgery
Department of Dentistry
Mount Sinai Hospital
Toronto, Ontario, Canada
Associate in Dentistry
Implant Prosthodontic Unit
Faculty of Dentistry
University of Toronto
Toronto, Ontario, Canada

**Steven E. Eckert**, DDS, MS
Professor
Division of Prosthodontics
Department of Dental Specialties
Mayo Medical School
Rochester, Minnesota

**Victoria Franke-Stenport**, DDS, PhD
Assistant Professor
Department of Biomaterials
Department of Prosthodontics
University of Gothenburg
Gothenburg, Sweden

**Sreenivas Koka**, DDS, MS, PhD
Professor and Chair
Division of Prosthodontics
Department of Dental Specialties
Mayo Medical School
Rochester, Minnesota

**ERNEST W. N. LAM**, DMD, PhD, FRCD(C)
Associate Professor
Department of Oral Radiology
Faculty of Dentistry
University of Toronto
Toronto, Ontario, Canada

**IAN R. MATTHEW**, BDS, MDentSc, PhD, FDSRCS
  (Eng/Edin)
Assistant Professor and Chair
Division of Oral and Maxillofacial Surgery
Department of Oral Biological and Medical Sciences
Faculty of Dentistry
University of British Columbia
Vancouver, British Columbia, Canada

**MICHAEL J. PHAROAH**, DDS, MSc, Dip Oral Rad,
  FRCD(C)
Professor and Head
Department of Oral Radiology
Faculty of Dentistry
University of Toronto
Toronto, Ontario, Canada

**KIRK PRESTON**, BSc, BEd, MEd, DDS, MSc
Prosthodontist
University of Toronto
Toronto, Ontario, Canada
Prosthodontist
Dalhousie University
Halifax, Nova Scotia, Canada

**DAVID J. PSUTKA**, DDS, FRCD(C)
Staff Surgeon
Division of Oral and Maxillofacial Surgery
Department of Dentistry
Mount Sinai Hospital
Toronto, Ontario, Canada
Associate in Dentistry
Oral and Maxillofacial Surgery and
  Implant Prosthodontic Unit
Faculty of Dentistry
University of Toronto
Toronto, Ontario, Canada

**CLARK STANFORD**, DDS, PhD
Associate Dean for Research
Centennial Fund Professor
College of Dentistry
University of Iowa
Iowa City, Iowa

**DENNIS P. TARNOW**, DDS
Professor and Chair
Department of Periodontology and Implant Dentistry
College of Dentistry
New York University
New York, New York

**ANN WENNERBERG**, DDS, PhD
Professor
Department of Biomaterials
University of Gothenburg
Gothenburg, Sweden
Professor
Department of Prosthodontics
University of Malmo
Malmo, Sweden

**CHRISTINE WHITE**, MA
Collegiate Librarian
College of Dentistry
University of Iowa
Iowa City, Iowa

**GEORGE A. ZARB**, BChD, DDS, MS, MS, FRCD(C)
Professor Emeritus
Department of Prosthodontics
Faculty of Dentistry
University of Toronto
Toronto, Ontario, Canada

# Looking Back: The Emergence and the Promise of Osseointegration

George A. Zarb

A frequently employed metaphor for modern life was first proposed by Marshall McLuhan (1911–1980), the late Canadian communications theorist. He described it as a journey undertaken in the automobile of progress—shiny new, fast, and replete with technological wonders—rushing forward at breakneck speed toward an undetermined horizon. He cautioned us as drivers never to lose sight of the rearview mirror or the surroundings, lest we forget the landscape we are driving through or where we are coming from. McLuhan's cautionary image is particularly relevant to health specialties such as dentistry, given the dominant influence of technology on its ongoing development.

This first chapter employs the metaphor to reflect the editors' perception of where we have been and where we are currently, in the context of osseointegration's impact on the management of partial and complete edentulism. Subsequent chapters sum up our convictions as to how far we have come and speculate on where we may be heading. We welcome readers to join us in the journey. We promise prudent speed and a more than cursory interpretative glance at the panorama we travel through.

Dental implants arguably have now eclipsed most traditional treatment topics as key practice interests in most clinical journals and meetings. This extraordinary therapeutic shift may be summarized in four general popular convictions:

1. Implants rarely fail and accompanying surgical morbidity is low and, if encountered, readily reversible through repeated surgical interventions.
2. Immediate loading of implants in virtually all jaw sites is routinely possible because of improvements in implant surface features and clinical handling.
3. Implant systems appear to be similar, and their diversity in microscopic and macroscopic design features is only necessary for commercial concerns.
4. Virtually all targeted host site implant locations can now be improved to ensure prognoses similar to those for native bone.

This clinical confidence reflects a remarkable shift in the profession's traditionally skeptical mind-set toward routine implant use. It was catalyzed by Brånemark's seminal research developments; virtually overnight, the notion of a reliable alloplastic analog for a tooth root and its attachment mechanism was matched with the repertoire of prosthodontic technology. Implants quickly assumed the status of a clinical panacea with provocative implications—an enlightened empiricism, a prevailing entrepreneurial spirit, and very aggressive marketing culture. Implant dentistry uniquely lent itself to the sort of clinical success that could now be purchased in a package. A new populist-driven treatment threshold had been crossed as the technique was recruited into dentistry's routine treatment repertoire.

In spite of these concerns, it is important to recall that most significant breakthroughs in clinical science resulted from unrelated but frequently convergent occurrences in the laboratory or at chairside. Small and often separate streams of thought from experiment and clinical application gradually merged to create a river, full of force and momentum, which in turn irrigated new sources of creativity. It is therefore desirable to look at the larger patient-need picture and endorse the current strong synergy of surgical and prosthodontic leadership and purpose in this field. It is also opportune—a quarter of a century after the introduction of osseointegration to North

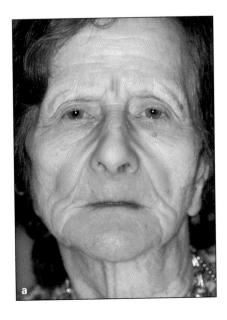
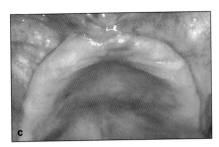
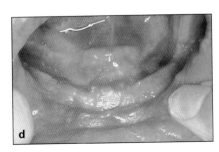
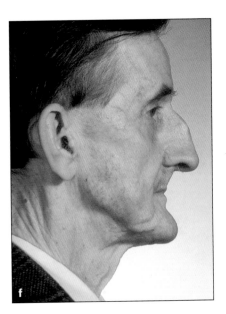
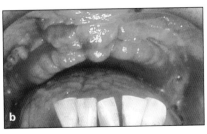
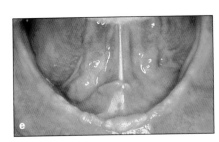

**Fig 1-1** *(a to f)* Adverse changes in intraoral and extraoral tissues over time are associated with denture wear.

America—to take stock of its documented effectiveness in the context of the rigorous documentation to improve and expand its applications. This is necessary to counter the competitive directives of commercial hype, which are rarely driven by exclusively patient- and dentist-mediated concerns.

This chapter reviews the implications of tooth loss, ecologic concerns in prosthodontic replacement, and the emergence of osseointegration as the standard therapeutic alternative.

## IMPLICATIONS OF TOOTH LOSS

While it is generally agreed that infective processes such as caries and periodontal disease are the exclusive cause of partial and complete edentulism, some authors argue that loss of teeth is unrelated to the prevalence of dental diseases. Both viewpoints are probably equally inaccurate, because current research underscores the role played by nondisease factors, such as the patient's attitude, behavior, and dental attendance, as well as the characteristics of available health care systems, in a patient's decision to allow extractions. In addition, a significant relationship appears to exist between personal economic concerns and low occupational levels—hence the general conclusion that tooth loss reflects cultural, financial, and dental disease attitudinal determinants, including perhaps a strong perception of treatment received in the past.

The heterogenous etiology of tooth loss has been addressed worldwide by the profession with a significantly reported decrease in the number of edentulous patients in industrial nations. Recent reviews of tooth loss and prevalence of edentulism in North America, Europe, Africa, and Australasia predict that treatment with complete dentures will continue to decline in the future, while the need for partially edentulous tooth replacements will increase, at least in the short term. While these predictions may suggest reduced numbers of patients with such needs, several significant concerns must be emphasized:

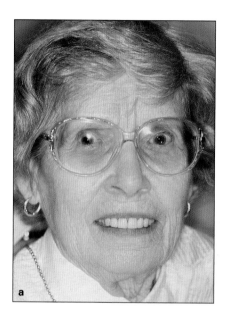
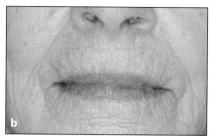
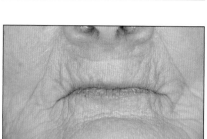
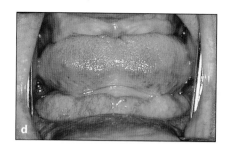
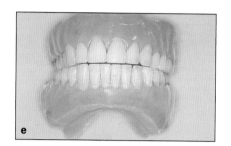
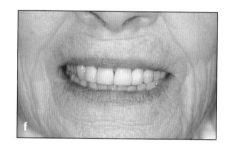

**Fig 1-2** *(a to d)* This octogenarian denture-wearer experienced deterioration and varying degrees of discomfort and dysfunction. *(e and f)* The progressive increase in the required bulk of her processed methyl methacrylate denture succeeded in alleviating her esthetic concerns. However, it proved a poor substitute for the missing quantitative and qualitative features of her absent periodontal ligament.

- Despite projections for tooth loss and edentulism in particular, the need for complete denture treatment is likely to continue at a high level.
- Predictions for the oral health status of healthy elderly individuals indicate that a high percentage will continue to be partially and completely edentulous. Consequently, the demand for tooth replacement in this cohort will remain high, and the need for acquisition of enhanced clinical skills will become an even more compelling professional practice concern.
- The implications of longevity's impact on tooth loss are still to be fully determined. However, clinical experience confirms that the cumulative consequences of both chronologic and biologic aging will confront dentists with an increased number of serious prosthodontic treatment challenges.

Irrespective of future patient needs and of the relationship between their chronology and systemic health, the psychologic and biomechanical consequences of tooth loss cannot be overlooked. Most patients regard loss of even a single tooth, especially if it is a visible one, as a minor mutilation and a strong incentive to seek dental care for its replacement. Loss of an entire dentition is even more dramatic and often regarded as the equivalent to the loss of a limb: a severe personal handicap. Dentists also regard tooth loss as posing the risk of age-dependent positional alterations in remaining tooth positions and the hazard of an even greater mutilation, namely the destruction of an integral part of the facial skeleton. Regrettably, the edentulous mouth is doomed to undergo adverse irreversible, variable, and severe morphologic changes with inevitable risks of esthetic and functional compromise (Figs 1-1 and 1-2).

Multiple to complete tooth loss imposes a varying degree of compromise of the masticatory system; affected individuals will perceive this compromise in different ways. Perceptions may range from feelings of inconvenience to ones of severe defect or abnormality. Although considerable research and emphasis have been devoted to the many forms of organ loss—mastectomies and hysterectomies for example—edentulism has received sparse psychologic attention. Only a few authors recognize its serious emotional implications, although

> **Box 1-1** Signs and Symptoms that may Preclude an Adaptive Complete Denture Experience
>
> - Severe morphologic compromise of the denture-supporting area that significantly undermines the retention of the denture
> - Poor oral muscular coordination
> - Low tolerance of the mucosal tissues
> - Unrealistic functional prosthodontic expectations
> - Parafunctional habits that lead to recurrent soreness and prosthetic instability
> - Active or hyperactive gag reflex elicited by wear of a removable prosthesis
> - Psychologic inability to wear a denture, even when adequate stability and retention are present

it is clearly not a life-threatening condition. This apparent lack of interest is probably the result of the relative prevalence of edentulism and the impressive success enjoyed by the dental profession in its management. Furthermore, edentulism is neither a disease nor a fatal condition; it has been shown to be an unlikely source of sympathy in a society preoccupied with youthful appearance.

Outcome measures of health care are also only partially defined by technical excellence and not exclusively dentist determined. Current scientific appraisals of treatment interventions and their outcomes seek to include patient perceptions, their responses to health care measures, and financial considerations in modern standards of health care evaluation.

It is important to recognize that even the prosthetically adaptive patient may eventually cross a functionally comfortable threshold into a future of denture-wearing problems. It is also significant to note that many patients who wear removable prostheses are actually unable to adapt to the experience. Alternatively they accept their predicament reluctantly, given the lack of a viable option.

These patients may be referred to as *prosthetically maladaptive*, a term we employ in this very specific context, because these individuals simply cannot adapt to wearing dentures in spite of their dentists' professional skills and compassion.

Box 1-1 lists factors that tend to preclude an adaptive experience. Dentists have persisted in their efforts to solve such patients' problems, convinced that they could compensate for conspicuous anatomic or physiologic challenges such as advanced residual ridge reduction, hyposalivation, or an acute gag reflex. In such situations, patients are treated with tech-

nique modifications or surgical attempts to enlarge the remaining denture-bearing areas, even if the initiatives have proven to be only palliative at best. Clinical experience has also shown that many patients who are initially prosthetically adaptive may end up as maladaptive (Fig 1-3). Time-dependent and regressive changes in the dentures' underlying support and accompanying neuromuscular control changes militate against a continuum of the expected functional and esthetic experience.

In fact, the entire field of prosthodontics (the removable component in particular) has suffered from an absence of methodologic rigor in developing defined treatment protocols and outcome measures to drive optimal clinical decisions. This is to a large extent understandable, given the dearth of alternative options for such patients. As a result, practical and useful studies involving presumed determinants of both patient- and dentist-mediated success, as well as quantifiable measurements of patients' quality of life after undergoing prosthodontic treatment, have underscored the relative unpredictability of complete denture service.

Some dissatisfied prosthesis-wearing patients become a source of anxiety for the profession and are all too readily dismissed as chronic complainers who must have some sort of personality disorder or cognitive dissonance and therefore need a psychiatrist or psychologist to solve their prosthodontic problem. The predicament these patients face often remains unsolved, a poignant reminder that no amount of perfectly processed and beautifully colored methyl methacrylate, supporting splendidly selected and arranged artificial teeth, would ever adequately substitute for a healthy periodontal ligament (PDL).

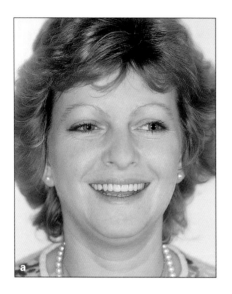
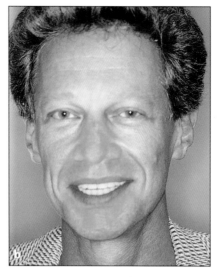
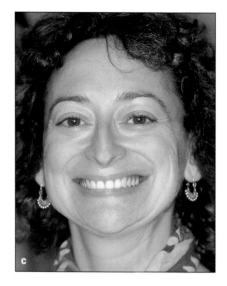

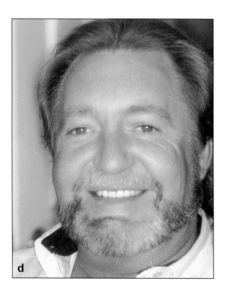
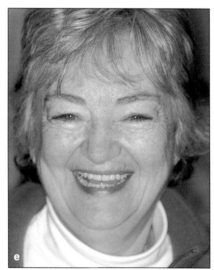
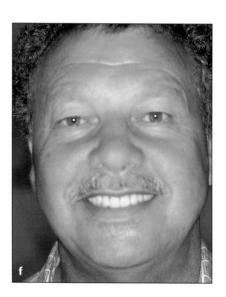

**Fig 1-3** Sex-paired examples of complete denture–wearers in their fourth *(a and b)*, fifth *(c and d)*, sixth *(e and f)*, and seventh *(g and h)* decades. All these patients started wearing complete dentures with initial adaptive prosthodontic experiences that eventually became maladaptive. They have now benefited immeasurably from new implant-supported prostheses.

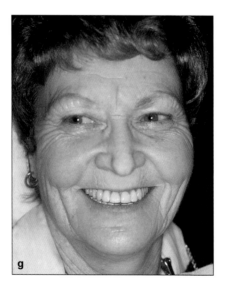
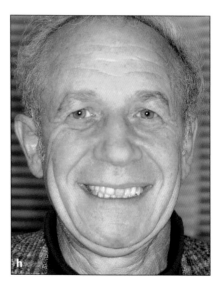

> **Box 1-2** FUNCTIONS OF THE PERIODONTAL
> LIGAMENT
>
> - Provides a viscoelastic cushion
> - Serves as a sensory organ
> - Accommodates tooth movements
> - Regulates osteogenesis

# ECOLOGIC CONCERNS IN PROSTHODONTIC TREATMENT

The mammalian periodontal ligament is a superbly evolved mechanism for the retention and support of the natural dentition (Box 1-2). It is quantitatively and qualitatively designed to cope with diverse and unpredictable magnitudes, durations, and frequencies of occlusal forces. It is, however, vulnerable to time-dependent sequelae of plaque accumulation. The latter plays a significant role in the pathogenesis of periodontal disease, which may in turn be affected by numerous systemic conditions, more especially if the latter are permitted to evolve to a brittle stage. However, it is generally agreed that in an infection-free environment the PDL will survive the life span of any individual.

The PDL has an approximate area of 45 cm$^2$ in each arch; with its inherent viscoelasticity and sophisticated sensory supply, the PDL ensures a built-in protective mechanism that virtually precludes traumatic damage from recurrent parafunctional overload and accompanying severe tooth damage (Fig 1-4). The PDL can also be clinically manipulated via controlled (contrived) light forces to induce safe movement of the dentition: hence, the ability to induce orthodontic tooth movement.

Should a hierarchy of qualitative functions be ranked, the most important functions of the healthy PDL are to permit osteogenesis regulation and ensure surrounding healthy bone. It is therefore not surprising that research observations have confirmed that, over the course of a lifetime, individuals with a healthy PDL will lose little vertical bone height around their dentitions. Moreover, even in the presence of variable amounts of bone loss, the clinician can reliably compensate for missing teeth and a consequent quantitative reduction of the total area of the dental arch by recruiting selected infection-free residual PDL for abutment support.

Appreciation for the PDL role must not preclude an understanding of dealing with its absence. The range of edentulous presentations demands much more than the automatic replacement of depleted "enamel units" with readily available synthetic mechanical and esthetic analogs for missing intraoral parts. It also demands an understanding of the inherent biologic risk that accompanies virtually all replacement interventions.

Adverse intraoral ecologic changes over time are virtually inevitable in prosthodontics. Given the unavailability of a PDL analog, past prosthetic support was provided by exclusive reliance on adjacent residual PDL (often already challenged by disease sequelae) or, worse, by residual ridge tissues with or without adjunctive PDL support. The concern regarding reliance on any amount of residual ridge area is its biomechanical inadequacy for providing long-term support for removable prostheses (Fig 1-5). Residual ridge tissues have been repeatedly shown to reduce in size over time. While the precise mechanism for such change is incompletely understood, it is presumed to be inevitable in a time-dependent context and also influenced by sex, age, load exposure, and systemic health conditions.

The implications of this tissue reduction are reflected in the realization that the edentulous maxilla and mandible offer 24 and 14 cm$^2$, respectively, of both quantitatively and qualitatively compromised support following tooth extractions (Fig 1-6). These compelling measurements are even more dramatic considering the inherent vulnerability of these residual areas and the fact that further reductions will ensue. These morphologic changes are inseparable from the qualitative changes implicit in the altered morphology.

Preprosthetic surgical interventions were developed to compensate for such compromise in the available stress-bearing edentulous areas. The major adjunctive treatment proposed for such patients usually involved enlargement of the denture-bearing areas by deepening labial, buccal, and sometimes even lingual vestibules or augmentation of entire residual ridge areas. Implicit in such surgical initiatives was the conviction that an enlarged denture-bearing area would increase the chances of denture stability and therefore patient adaptation. The procedures were not without their risks of morbidity, including donor site problems, altered sensation, and pain. However, the major lingering concern was their longitudinal unpredictability and the ongoing risk of additional changes in the prosthesis-bearing tissue support.

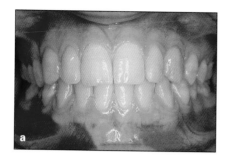
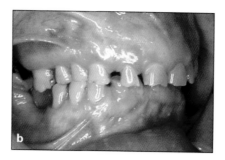
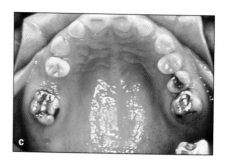

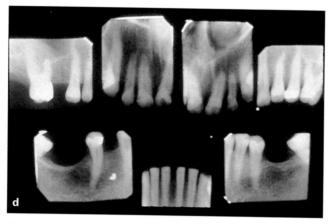

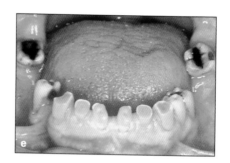

**Fig 1-4** *(a)* The average area of periodontal ligament in each dental arch is 45 cm². *(b to e)* The ligament appears capable of enduring a vast range of occlusal forces without compromise as long as no infective process is present. The sequence of illustrations reconciles the clinical display of severe tooth wear with radiographic evidence of healthily maintained supporting bone. *(f)* Prosthodontic management can compensate for even severe deficits in the periodontal ligament area, such as that pictured here.

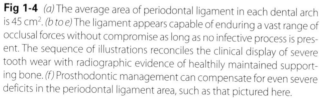

**Fig 1-5** *(a to d)* A range of periodontal ligament deficits is illustrated, wherein variable areas of tooth loss are replaced by residual alveolar ridges. Treatment strategies for these dentitions could include recognition of the merits of the shortened dental arch, removable or fixed implant-supported interventions, and even extractions to permit a complete-arch implant-supported fixed or overdenture replacement.

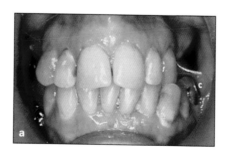
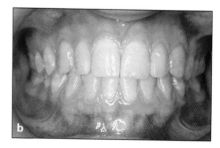

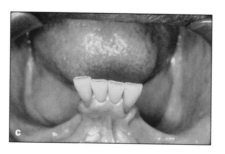
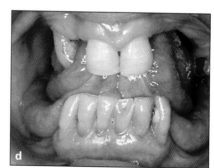

7

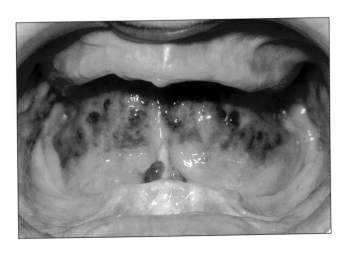

**Fig 1-6** These edentulous arches offer a significantly compromised support area for a prosthetic occlusion—reduced from 45 cm$^2$ of periodontal ligament in each arch to 24 cm$^2$ in the maxilla and 14 cm$^2$ in the mandible. These areas of mucoperiosteum and underlying alveolar bone also offer qualitatively poor long-term occlusal load-bearing potential in the context of prolonged wear of removable prostheses.

It is prudent to highlight concerns regarding the efficacy and effectiveness of any routine treatment plan with two key questions:

1. What are the biologic, mechanical, and esthetic sequelae of tooth loss?
2. What are the biologic or morbidity risks inherent to any selected intervention?

Answers to both questions underscore the objective of best-evidence clinical decision making.

# EMERGENCE OF OSSEOINTEGRATION

Per-Ingvar Brånemark's seminal research linked diverse biologic facts and observations into a coherent whole. He coined the term *osseointegration* for his proposed surgical and loading protocols. This concept resulted in a biologic outcome that is now widely regarded as a breakthrough in the management of partial and complete edentulism.

There have been numerous attempts to define osseointegration. The clinically convenient current definition is: *a time-dependent healing process whereby clinically asymptomatic rigid fixation of specifically designed alloplastic materials is achieved and maintained during functional loading* (Figs 1-7 and 1-8). The application of osseointegration catalyzed rapid advances in preprosthetic surgery, applied dental biotechnology, and an entire spectrum of prosthodontic applications. Above all, it

introduced an entirely new standard of patient- and dentist-mediated expectations for treatment outcomes. The method has now become an integral part of the routine treatment repertoire for most dentists and is rapidly acquiring an important place in dental educational curricula.

Traditional protocols combined with prosthodontic and surgical virtuosity permitted solutions to many complex rehabilitation problems in the past. However, scenarios such as so-called periodontal prostheses (much loved by "herodontists" in specialty groups) were long on anecdote if short on scientific veracity. They were daring and technically impressive efforts to prolong the useful life of an already seriously depleted PDL and demanded considerable technical and clinical skills. They were also expensive, and their beneficial outcomes were frequently transient. These well-intentioned efforts highlighted the lengths patients and professionals would go to in order to avoid the need for dentures (Fig 1-9).

In the pre-Brånemark era, dental journals and meetings were dominated by technique and dental materials presentations, and prospective clinical outcome studies were rarely encountered. The rigor implicit in currently accepted principles of clinical epidemiology was conspicuously absent, even if the need for prudent analyses of treatment results was regularly acknowledged.

The bottom line in everyday practice was a fine-tuned hierarchy of interventions, a commonsense decision-making process that reconciled clinical skill, laboratory support availability, patient input and appreciation, and financial considerations. What was conspicuously absent from daily practice was a predictable analog for the periodontal ligament to simplify and optimize treatment plans. It is therefore plausible to regard the entire pre-osseointegration era as one of the treatment meth-

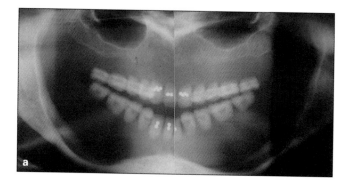
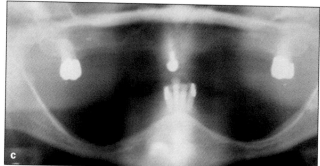
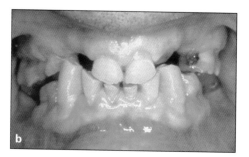
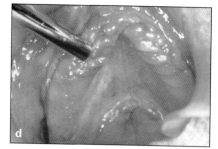
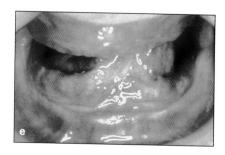

**Fig 1-7** *(a to e)* A likely result of long-term prosthesis-wearing experience and occlusal trauma is damage to the prosthesis-support area.

ods in search of a unifying conceptual principle regarding support for a replaced dentition. Consequently the notion of endosseous implants (numerous designs manufactured out of different alloys and employing nonspecific surgical protocols) evolved slowly. The resulting unpredictable nature of the induced interface was invariably an inherent flaw. Brånemark's research revolutionized the approach and provided an application of the desired conceptual principle (Figs 1-10 to 1-12). The therapeutic breakthrough, from a clinical standpoint, was a scientific transition from an uncontrolled to a controlled interface. With this technique, the nature of the interface at a microscopic level can be compared to a biologic "Velcro-type" response, which presumably can be further enhanced via controlled roughening of the surface of the alloplastic material.

The following attempt to summarize the current status of applied osseointegration underscores the subtle yet often profound contrasts that are encountered in patients with different types of complete and partial edentulism, periodontal disease of dubious prognosis, or maxillofacial deficits.

## Management of complete edentulism

The esthetic and biomechanical consequences of loss of the entire PDL compromise the potential support for any planned prostheses, because residual ridges are such a poor substitute. Complete denture therapy has focused largely on clinical judgment combined with technical and interpersonal skills. This approach nurtured the development of new techniques and materials plus an understanding of the relationships among esthetics, occlusion, and patient expectations. Strong convictions about treatment results led dentists to presume that their clinical endeavors fell just short of the gold standard of a healthy intact dentition.

Most denture-wearing patients clearly benefited from this professional commitment and even influenced other patients with compromised oral health to select extractions and complete denture replacement, rather than undergo the required necessary extensive (and often expensive) periodontal and restorative treatments to preserve teeth. Regrettably this approach

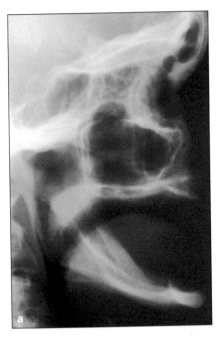

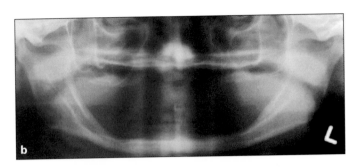

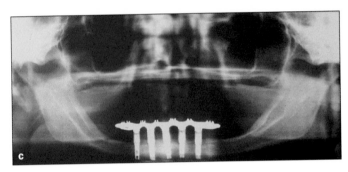

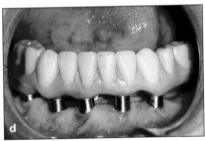

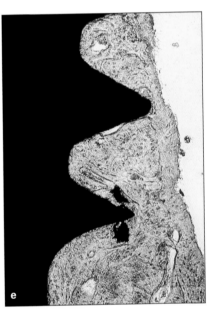

**Fig 1-8** Osseointegrated implant support and retention for a fixed prosthesis in an edentulous mandibular arch *(a to d)* results from a controlled interfacial healing response *(e)*.

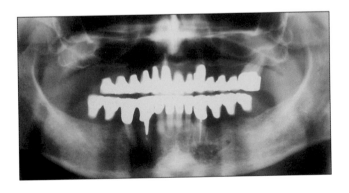

**Fig 1-9** This particular herodontic approach involved the ingenious, if tenuous, exploitation of residual periodontal ligament for fixed prosthodontic management. Very long-span fixed partial dentures were designed in both arches in an effort to harness the qualitative and quantitative aspects of an area severely depleted of abutment support. This so-called periodontal prosthesis treatment plan was rapidly eclipsed by osseointegration-based strategies.

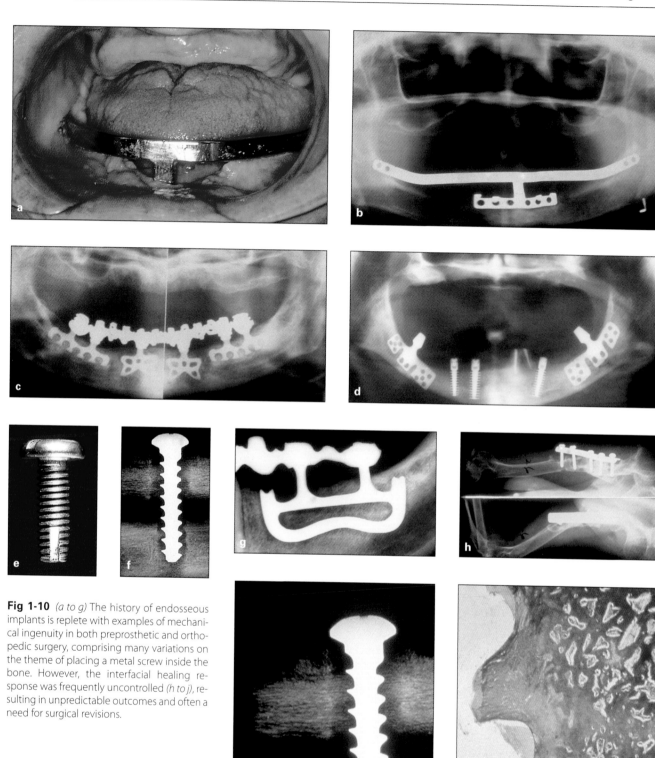

**Fig 1-10** *(a to g)* The history of endosseous implants is replete with examples of mechanical ingenuity in both preprosthetic and orthopedic surgery, comprising many variations on the theme of placing a metal screw inside the bone. However, the interfacial healing response was frequently uncontrolled *(h to j)*, resulting in unpredictable outcomes and often a need for surgical revisions.

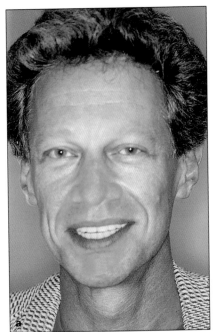
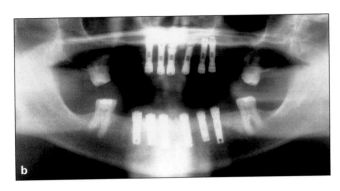
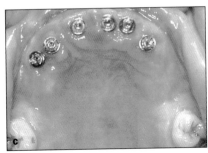
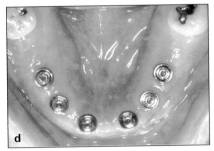

**Fig 1-11** *(a to d)* The introduction of the osseointegration concept resulted in the development of predictable and long-lasting methods to replace an entire missing dentition.

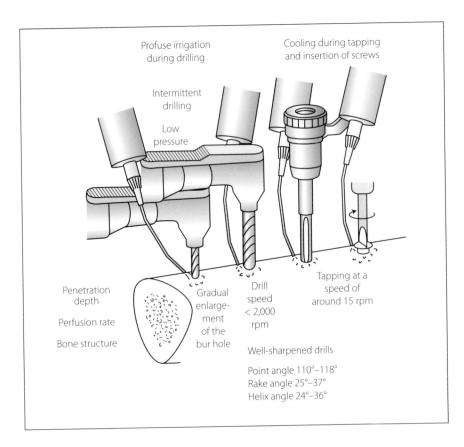

Profuse irrigation during drilling

Cooling during tapping and insertion of screws

Intermittent drilling

Low pressure

Penetration depth

Perfusion rate

Bone structure

Gradual enlarge-ment of the bur hole

Drill speed < 2,000 rpm

Tapping at a speed of around 15 rpm

Well-sharpened drills

Point angle 110°–118°
Rake angle 25°–37°
Helix angle 24°–36°

**Fig 1-12** The success of osseointegration resulted primarily from the original scrupulous surgical protocol that still underlies today's methods. Note that developments in self-tapping implants now preclude the need for tapping the implant site. (Modified from Eriksson[1] with permission.)

**Fig 1-13** The use of two or more abutments to stabilize, and indeed retain, a mandibular removable overdenture rapidly became a viable alternative to the fixed implant solution for prosthodontically maladaptive edentulous patients. It is now routine to offer the approach to both newly edentulous patients *(a)* as well as those who had resorted to earlier preprosthetic surgical interventions *(b)*, such as a mandibular sulcus deepening with a skin graft, to address their denture-wearing problems.

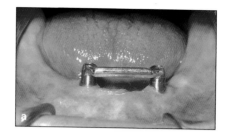 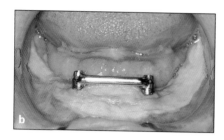

was also followed by some individuals whose dissatisfaction with the appearance of their natural teeth could also be addressed by converting to a complete denture to achieve a better appearance.

There is little doubt that the complete denture era of education and treatment did contribute to a better quality of life for most edentulous patients. In a public health context, complete dentures remain a relatively simple and inexpensive treatment method, one that offers scope for virtual universal application. Moreover, as a clinical teaching tool, the protocol demands knowledge of applied basic sciences, biomaterials, and occlusion and provides the challenge and satisfaction of managing patients' behavioral and age-related concerns and infirmities. It also remains the basis for most current esthetic clues or decisions to improve and create natural smiles.

The osseointegration method was originally introduced for edentulous patients. The first successful Swedish trials of the technique were compellingly replicated in several teaching centers and private practices around the world. The published results comprise some of the best long-term scientifically documented evidence for any therapeutic dental procedure. This fact is particularly significant when viewed in the context of biologic and chronologic changes in the population. The luxury of aging was one of the major achievements of the 20th century, resulting from a miracle medicine scenario that has been now augmented with new promises of genetic engineering and regenerative medicine.

Dentistry has successfully addressed sequelae of oral disease and in the process also provided orofacial "spare parts". This was achieved without the need for dealing with tricky ethical questions such as the agonizing ones that hallmarked medical breakthroughs in genetics and organ transplantation. In fact the claim for the evidence-based biotechnology of osseointegration reached its apogee almost three decades ago. Today, comprehensive clinical research endorses the benefits of implant-supported and -retained partial or complete prostheses. The aged edentulous patient, particularly if burdened

with denture adaptation problems, need no longer suffer. Nor is such a predicament imposed on any patient who no longer wants to wear a removable prosthesis.

The introduction of osseointegration catalyzed an entirely new dimension for management of the edentulous condition. The controlled change in the nature of support ensured stable prostheses and the desired sense of security and well-being that most denture-wearers never realized could be regained. As a result, all edentulous patients can now be routinely offered three treatment options for the management of their condition: complete dentures or the choice between an implant-supported and -retained fixed denture and a removable overdenture (Fig 1-13).

The best option is not always clear because the clinical decision should reflect the dentist's knowledge of efficacy and effectiveness outcomes as well as the patient's understanding of attendant risks and the cost-effectiveness of the technique. Biologic, functional, personality, and fiscal concerns may also preclude one option or another. The traditional complete denture lends itself to a relatively routine clinical protocol if costs are a major determinant of the patient's choice. It may very well be the opportune treatment until a patient is prepared to move to the next treatment consideration with its accompanying advantages.

The implant-supported overdenture has now been shown to rectify most maladaptive concerns, because the major complaint of denture instability is readily solved. It is also easier to keep clean, particularly where caregivers are the sole providers of the required hygiene service. Implant-supported overdentures also offer optimal esthetic results when severe morphologic soft tissue deficits are encountered. The method can be regarded as combining the better of two techniques: a stable prosthesis-wearing experience without the considerable expense of a fixed implant-supported restoration. It is therefore reasonable to suggest that the optimal management of edentulism for maladaptive patients should also include consideration of an implant-supported prescription.

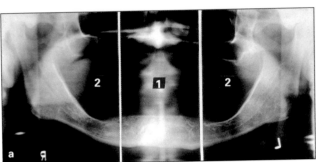 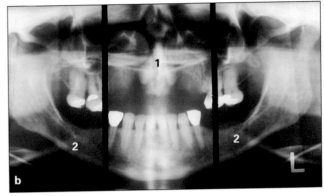

**Fig 1-14** In both edentulous (a) and partially edentulous (b) patients, subtle or profound differences that exist in host bone sites may be differentiated by arbitrary vertical lines drawn at right angles to the mental foramina on the panoramic radiograph. The resultant anterior (1) and posterior (2) zones permit considerations of anatomic landmarks, host site dimensions, occlusal considerations, and esthetics to influence prosthetic designs.

## Management of partial edentulism

The trajectory of successful management of edentulism rapidly led to application of implants to partially edentulous patients. The ease and predictability of PDL replacement resulted from a protocol identical to the one employed in the edentulous patient (Figs 1-14 and 1-15). It was largely a lateral move in skill application, although additional specific determinants demanded some variations in the decision-making protocol.

A proposed estimate of differences encountered in bone quantity and quality is described in the surgical and prosthodontic chapters. It resulted in a working classification that proved to be a useful starting point for treatment planning for most edentulous patients (Fig 1-16).

The scope of the classification was readily expanded to include the posterior edentulous sites where implants would also now have to be routinely placed. Surgically challenging quantitative concerns in these sites would prove to be more critical given the variable restrictions imposed by the position of the inferior alveolar canal and its contents in the posterior mandible and of the maxillary sinus in the posterior maxilla. These often tricky morphologic features, coupled with more challenging bone quality concerns, demanded more rigorous imaging of the proposed host sites together with even more rigorous surgical skills.

A similar challenge was the nature of the esthetic result, because management of anterior partial edentulism frequently required more difficult decisions, skills, and techniques than either posterior replacement or complete edentulism (Figs 1-17 to 1-21). Additional concerns included the realization that acute force development in the posterior zones would be likely to be more severe, especially in the context of a fewer number of and even shorter implants recruited for proposed abutment service.

As a result, a treatment planning formula evolved that included specific and very accurate site imaging, selection of the maximum number and size of implants perceived as suitable for their assigned abutment role and within the available area for their location, a patient-customized occlusal and esthetic strategy, and the necessary surgical decision as to how to modify the site to ensure an optimal result. Well-documented treatment outcomes are now available for both anterior and posterior edentulous sites with impressively favorable results, permitting an expanded and even more versatile application of the technique.

The development of osseointegration from edentulous management to partially edentulous treatment resulted from the method's three irrefutable achievements: scope for stable and retentive prosthesis support, retardation of residual ridge reduction, and minimal risk of preprosthetic surgical morbidity. Furthermore, the induced ankylotic-like response revealed a very important difference from the PDL, which is the result of a *developmental phenomenon*. In contrast, the implant's bony attachment results from an *induced healing response*.

Consequently, the small number of reported implant failures during the prescribed healing interval when a two-stage surgical procedure is used may result from a compromised healing response. Other failures may also occur after loading of the implants (so-called late failures), but the premise is that the healing was compromised in the first place and therefore vulnerable to relative overload over time. In addition, such a flawed interface may be vulnerable to infection, which will then become a secondary superimposed insult. This suggests that the pathogenesis of induced osseointegration attachment failure may be very different from the pathogenesis of chronic periodontal disease. This difference has significant treatment planning implications. This topic is discussed further in chapter 11.

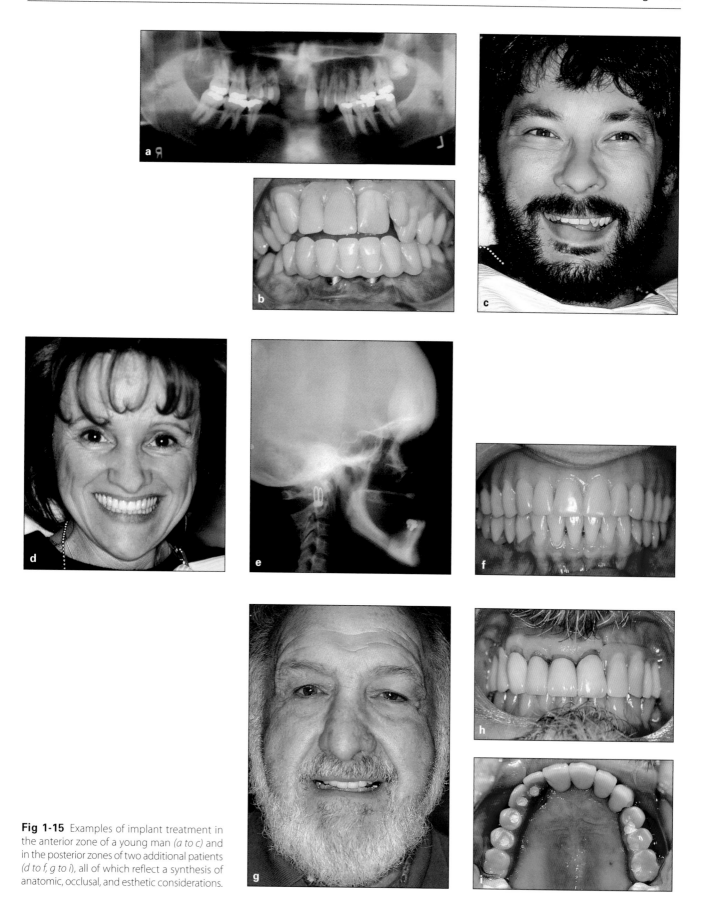

**Fig 1-15** Examples of implant treatment in the anterior zone of a young man (a to c) and in the posterior zones of two additional patients (d to f, g to i), all of which reflect a synthesis of anatomic, occlusal, and esthetic considerations.

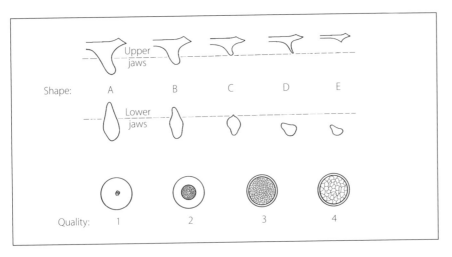

**Fig 1-16** The proposed working classification of bone quantity and quality in edentulous patients proved to be a useful starting point for determining the numbers and sizes of implants prescribed for anterior sites. (Reprinted from Lekholm and Zarb[2] with permission.)

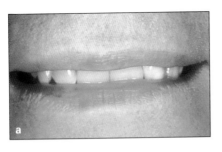
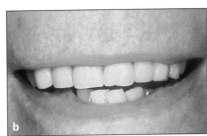
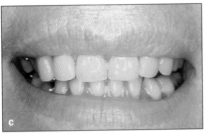
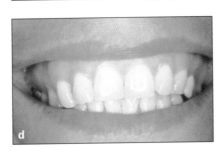

**Fig 1-17** (a to d) Partial edentulism in the anterior zone demands scrutiny of the patient's smile line and circumoral range of activities.

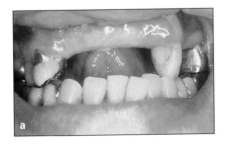
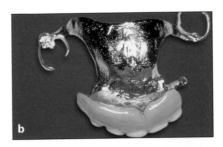

**Fig 1-18** (a to d) Versatile esthetic support from labial flanges must be considered, even when fixed prostheses are prescribed.

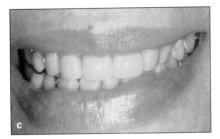
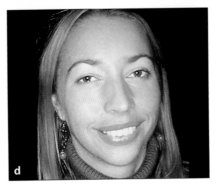

**Fig 1-19** *(a and b)* A range of implant-supported prosthetic solutions is possible in the context of different smiles. Here, circumoral smiling activity does not expose the relationship between the prosthetic pontics and the altered gingival morphologic features. Compare the clinical result achieved with those shown in Figs 1-20 and 1-21.

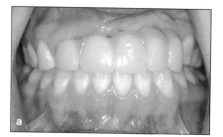

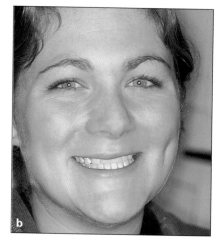

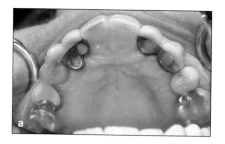

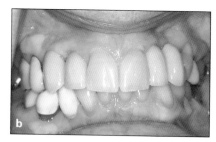

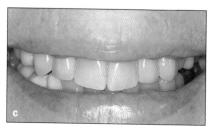

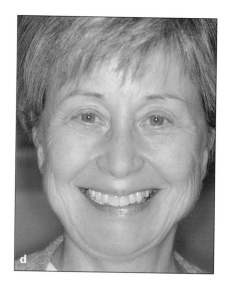

**Fig 1-20** *(a to d)* Bilateral implant-supported fixed replacements make for well-designed pontic relationships to both underlying and overlying soft tissues.

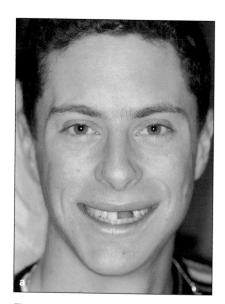

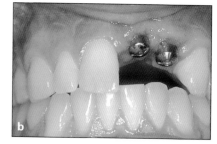

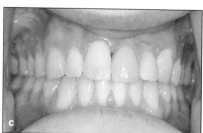

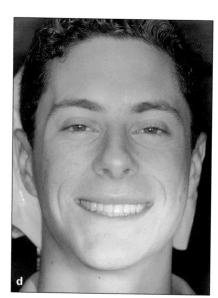

**Fig 1-21** *(a to d)* The same principles as in Figs 1-19 and 1-20 apply to the prosthodontic design employed for this young male patient whose anterior teeth and part of the supporting bone were avulsed in a traumatic accident.

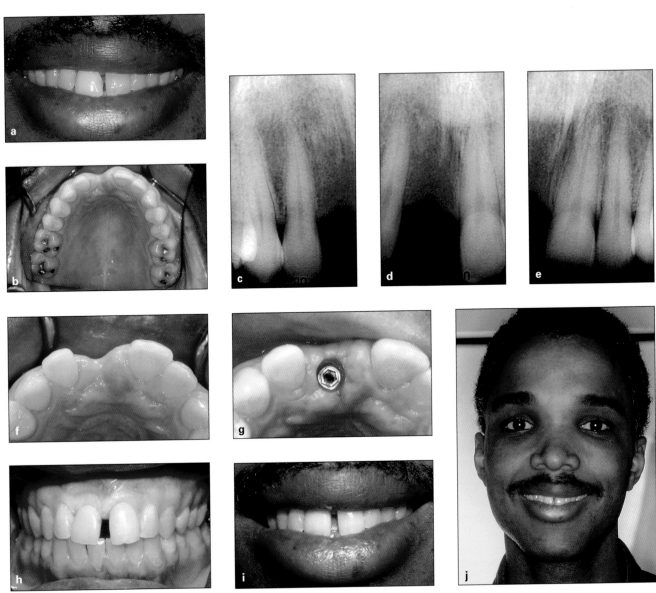

**Fig 1-22** *(a to e)* Prosthodontic design skills must be reconciled with scrupulous evaluation of residual peri-implant soft tissues. In this patient the missing tooth and cervical alveolar tissues do not affect space requirements for implant placement. However, they create the need for serious consideration of the replacement tooth's emergence profile if an esthetic result is to be ensured. *(f to h)* In this clinical situation, the depth and distension potential of the soft tissue at the implant's bony site location permitted "plumping" of the subgingival cervical porcelain crown. This decision precluded the need for a surgical procedure to surgically augment the labial gingival tissue. *(i and j)* It is important to appreciate the fact that the outcome of any surgical intervention does not guarantee a perfect esthetic result.

Replacement of a missing single tooth in either the anterior or posterior zones with an osseointegrated implant is inarguably a most ecologically prudent prosthodontic intervention. However, most situations in the anterior zone present specific esthetic challenges. These may be dominant concerns if generous smile morphology is present, particularly if the residual soft tissue support requires compensation (Fig 1-22). When bone deficits are present they are frequently and routinely compensated for by the skillful use of autogenous or even alloplastic grafts; minor bone deficits may be eliminated through regenerative protocols. However, this is not always

the case with soft tissue deficits. Their reported management tends to make for exciting presentations, but it remains dominated by anecdotal-type evidence (see chapter 8).

## Management of periodontal disease with poor prognosis

Chronic periodontitis is an inflammatory disease of the periodontal ligament caused by specific pathogens and resulting in progressive bone loss around the dentition. Its management

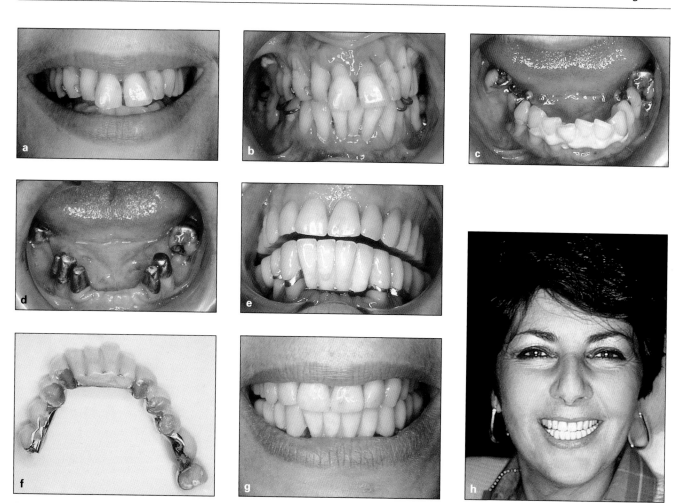

**Fig 1-23** *(a to h)* Before the osseointegration era, clinical ingenuity and a serious lack of standardized outcome criteria characterized the approach to prolonging the useful life of a few abutments for prosthodontic service. These images of one particular case history illustrate this point. The residual and severely compromised dentition was managed via selective extractions and a provisional splint in anticipation of a sequenced placement of implants.

is largely dependent on a diligent program of self-managed and sustained plaque control, in addition to professional supportive measures to facilitate the patient's efforts to control the infection. These measures include related and modifiable environmental and behavioral initiatives, especially in the areas of smoking, stress, and endocrine disorders such as diabetes.

Current research has targeted efforts to identify subject-, tooth-, or even site-specific factors that may predict or guide a research-driven approach to outcomes of protocols for infection control. There have also been reports on numerous mechanical and biologic mediators to support the recovery of lost attachment around teeth. As a result, chronic periodontal disease is no longer regarded as an inevitable precursor of edentulism. Nonetheless, affected patients may opt for a treatment approach of extractions and implants as an alternative to disciplining themselves to the rigors of long-term periodontal therapy. Noncompliance or, more frequently, an unfavorable prognosis has now become a strong incentive for the dentist

to offer the implant treatment alternative. This approach is meant to reduce the adverse impact on bone maintenance in the presence of an active disease condition. Furthermore, a recent report has also demonstrated that complete-mouth extractions actually lower systemic inflammatory and thrombotic markers of cardiovascular risk.

The implant option expanded the treatment choice repertoire for patients with chronic periodontal disease. As a result, today's disease management options may depend on much more than an evidence-based prognosis for an individual patient's periodontal disease management. Other considerations include expected discomfort and pain, apprehension, root sensitivity, esthetic and phonetic considerations, and time-dependent expenses incurred. Furthermore, the osseointegration technique permits a versatile approach to managing the predicament of advanced periodontal disease, because overall treatment can be staged in a manner that reconciles most patient-mediated concerns (Fig 1-23).

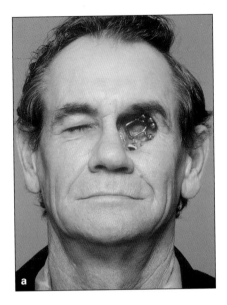
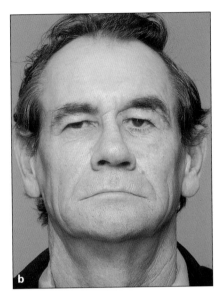

**Fig 1-24** *(a and b)* Osseointegration virtually revolutionized the prosthodontic management of maxillofacial patients, as shown for a patient with an orbital prosthesis. (Courtesy of Dr James D. Anderson, University of Toronto.)

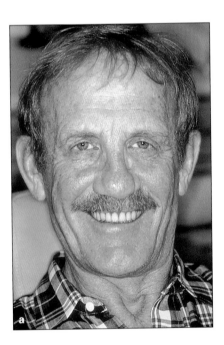
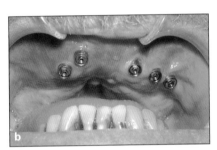
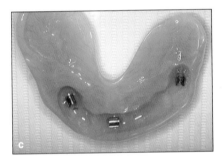

**Fig 1-25** *(a to c)* Adult cleft palate patient with a maxillary overdenture.

## Management of maxillofacial defects

Orofacial trauma, congenital anomalies, and surgical treatment of malignancies often result in significantly compromised anatomic structures. This is a serious challenge for the prosthodontist who seeks to provide a functional and esthetic reconstruction for patients while attempting to satisfy criteria similar to those for traditional intraoral prostheses. For many years this undertaking was undermined by difficulties with prosthetic retention, impaired tongue function, varying degrees of neutral zone reduction, and severely compromised soft and hard tissue load-bearing areas.

Implant-supported and -retained prostheses have been increasingly prescribed for such patients, providing extraordinary advances in treatment outcomes (Figs 1-24 to 1-27). The validation of such interventions is not an easy research task, although individual patient responses support the premise that patients' quality of life is profoundly and positively influenced by the adjunctive role of implants in current overall treatment planning. These successes represent an endorsement of the role of osseointegration in the expansion of the dentist's therapeutic repertoire.

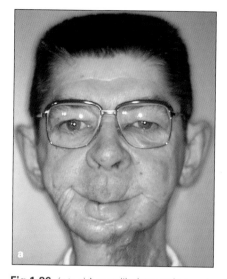
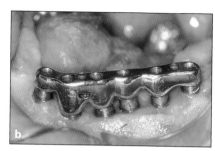
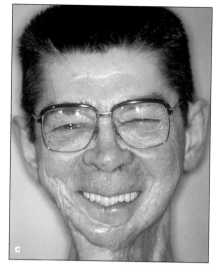

**Fig 1-26** *(a to c)* A mandibular overdenture has been modified to improve speech, given the nature of the resected mandible and tongue.

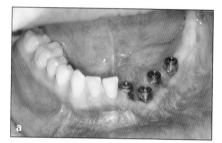
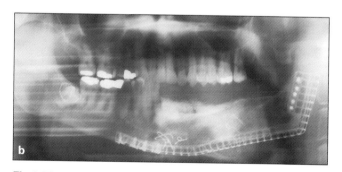
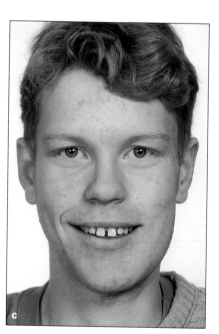

**Fig 1-27** *(a to c)* A fixed mandibular prosthesis has replaced the dental quadrant in a young man after a mandibular resection with grafted restoration of the mandible's continuity.

# REFERENCES

1. Eriksson AR. Heat-Induced Bone Injury. An In Vivo Investigation of Heat Tolerance of Bone Tissue and Temperature Rise in Drilling of Cortical Bone [thesis]. Gothenburg, Sweden: University of Gothenburg, 1984.
2. Lekholm U, Zarb GA. Patient selection and preparation. In: Brånemark P-I, Zarb GA, Albrektsson T (eds). Tissue-Integrated Prostheses: Osseointegration in Clinical Dentistry. Chicago: Quintessence, 1985:199–209.

# RECOMMENDED READING

Laney WR. State of the Science on Implant Dentistry: Consensus Conference Proceedings. J Oral Maxillofac Implants 2007;22(suppl):1–226.
Taylor BA, Tofler GH, Carey HM, et al. Full-mouth tooth extraction lowers systemic inflammatory and thrombotic markers of cardiovascular risk. J Dent Res 2006;85:74–78.
Zarb GA, MacEntee M, Anderson JD (eds). On biological and social interfaces in prosthodontics: Proceedings of an international symposium. Int J Prosthodont 2003;16(suppl):1–94.

# Treatment Outcomes

George A. Zarb | Tomas Albrektsson

The currency of success in implant treatment may be regarded as a therapeutic coin. One side of the coin comprises the controllable physical aspects of macroscopic and microscopic implant design features, including the selected alloplastic material. The other side involves the patient's biologic reactions as mediated by the health professional's judgment and skill. Both sides can be analyzed and researched separately, but, ultimately, successfully predictable outcomes will only result from a convergence of the clinical certainties of treatment prudence, professional integrity, and scrupulous documentation.

## Determinants for Success

The six parameters described in Box 2-1 are widely regarded as key determinants for successful osseointegration. When employed synergistically, they produce an interface that consists mainly of bone tissue—a clinically asymptomatic rigid anchorage of the tooth root analogs in bone. This biologic phenomenon depends on the unique self-repairing ability of a surgically prepared bony interface. If the healing process is not unduly disturbed, bone remodels sufficiently to carry clinical loads. This is certainly not the case when a soft tissue interface develops as a result of compromised healing; the latter interfacial outcome leads to unpredictable clinical results in contrast to those recorded for a bone-implant surface.

It is tempting, indeed logical, to reconcile measurable implant–bone surface contact with successful long-term os-

seointegration. After all, implant choice, optimal imaging, and site selection, coupled with surgical skill, aim at implant stability via maximum bone contact and ingrowth (Figs 2-1 and 2-2 and Table 2-1). Achievement of this goal, coupled with a recorded, quantifiable figure for the number of implant units recruited into prosthesis support, could then predict the amount of occlusal loading the induced interface could sustain under adverse long-term loading conditions. This premise could then be reconciled further with age- and disease-related changes in bone as well as the range of forces implicit in the different magnitudes and durations of the imposed occlusal forces.

Regrettably, this type of detailed analysis has not been the case, and the routine prescription of more, longer, wider, and rougher-surfaced implants tends to be the automatic reaction to treatment planning. These measures are certainly not imprudent, but the loading limits of a single successfully osseointegrated implant in different jawbone sites, in the context of age and health and their many variations, remain imperfectly understood. Nonetheless, the well-documented longitudinal success of the initial Brånemark formula (Fig 2-3) has permitted versatile treatment extrapolations with impressive reported results for different sites and in different age groups (Figs 2-4 to 2-9).

In addition, even imaged unfavorable differences in bone quality are no longer regarded as unequivocal contraindications for implant placement. For example, osteoporosis-like bone characterized by cortical porosity and trabecular disruption has been convincingly reported as a viable site for implant placement if the planned surgical and loading pro-

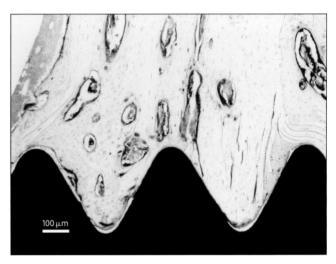

**Fig 2-1** Histologic depiction of an area of host bone-implant interface. It is presumed that a predictable and controlled expansion of this interface provides the desired holding power required to support diverse prosthetic designs.

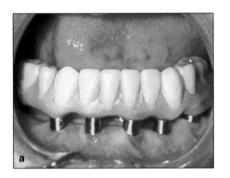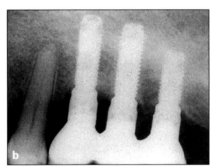

**Fig 2-2** Diverse surface areas are required for different abutment dimensions. For example, relatively abbreviated support (5 × 10–mm implants) is required for a complete mandibular arch rehabilitation *(a)* while a maxillary posterior sextant opposing a natural or a restored fixed dentition appears to require as much support as possible (in this case three implants of different lengths as determined by available host bone height) *(b)*.

tocols are suitably modified. Hence osteoporosis per se is not an outright contraindication for implant placement (see chapter 3).

The ongoing and remarkable adaptive capacity of bone takes place in accordance with an individual's systemic health status in the context of imposed and time-dependent occlusal loads and results in a biomechanical bond over the surface of the osseointegrated implant. The resulting bond appears to have the potential for indefinite maintenance throughout a patient's lifetime, irrespective of fluctuations in health.

A short description of the cited parameters will facilitate an appreciation of the more extensive analyses in other chapters, as indicated in Box 2-1.

## Implant biocompatibility

The most commonly used intraosseous materials in dentistry are commercially pure titanium and titanium alloys. Both demonstrate excellent in vitro and in vivo tissue reactions, and their routine clinical use is now endorsed by numerous studies. The former remains the best documented material from a hard tissue response point of view, while a recent consensus conference literature review concluded that it is also the only material with a proven soft tissue biocompatibility (see chapter 5). However, good data supporting the merits of using titanium-6 aluminum-4 vanadium are also available. It may be difficult to assign clinical significance to the

TABLE 2-1   SURFACE AREA OF IMPLANTS*

| Implant size (mm) | Bone contact area (mm²) | Threaded area (mm²) | Threaded length (mm) |
|---|---|---|---|
| 3.75 × 7.00 | 102 | 67 | 4.0 |
| 3.75 × 10.00 | 166 | 119 | 7.0 |
| 3.75 × 13.00 | 224 | 170 | 10.0 |
| 3.75 × 15.00 | 264 | 204 | 12.0 |
| 3.75 × 18.00 | 315 | 255 | 15.0 |
| 3.75 × 20.00 | 350 | 290 | 17.0 |
| 5.00 × 6.00 | 139 | 102 | 4.5 |
| 5.00 × 8.00 | 185 | 136 | 6.0 |
| 5.00 × 10.00 | 231 | 170 | 7.5 |
| 5.00 × 12.00 | 276 | 204 | 9.0 |

*Dimensional values of a particular threaded implant as based on information supplied by its manufacturer.

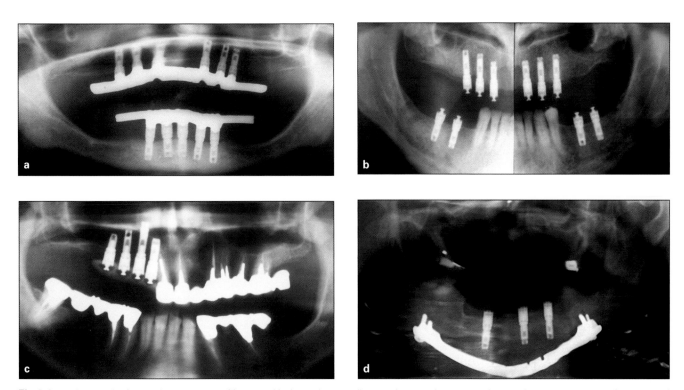

**Fig 2-3** (a) The initial Brånemark prescription of five mandibular and six maxillary implants, each 10.00 mm long and 3.75 to 4.00 mm in diameter and supporting fixed prostheses, yielded compellingly documented and favorable long-term clinical outcomes. This formula was rapidly adopted for numerous partially edentulous posterior zones (b and c) as well as for a range of grafted sites (d).

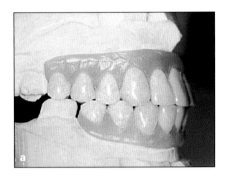 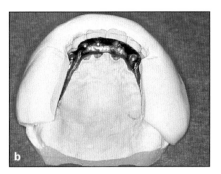

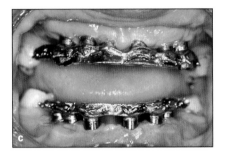 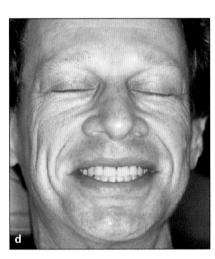

**Fig 2-4** The osseointegration technique shows great clinical versatility. *(a to d)* In this case, it allowed fixed prosthodontic management of several congenitally missing maxillary and mandibular teeth in a middle-aged man. All four second molars were present and retained to ensure a stable vertical dimension of occlusion while the patient wore provisional removable prostheses.

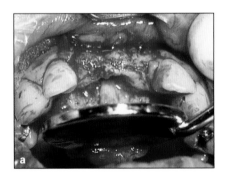 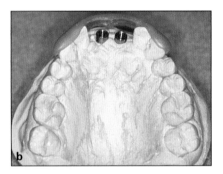

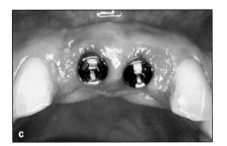 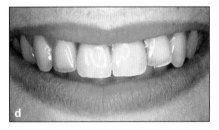

**Fig 2-5** *(a to d)* Maxillary implants are placed to support fixed replacements for Kennedy Class IV partial edentulism in a patient with a favorable smile line.

**Fig 2-6** Mandibular implants are placed to support a fixed restoration in a patient with Kennedy Class IV partial edentulism. *(a and b)* The customized gold alloy casting is tried on the two implants. The final result is demonstrated with cheek retractors in place *(c)* and in the presence of favorable circumoral smile activity *(d)*.

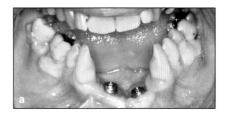

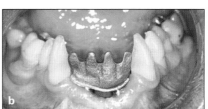

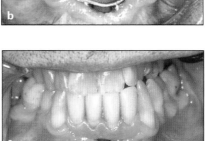

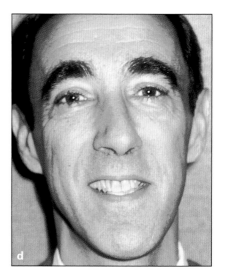

**Fig 2-7** Anodontia in a young woman is managed with selective extractions and preprosthetic orthodontic treatment followed by placement of implant-supported fixed prostheses. The series of pictures demonstrates the esthetic result obtained both intraorally *(a to c)* and extraorally *(d and e)* .

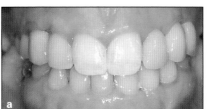

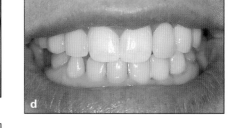

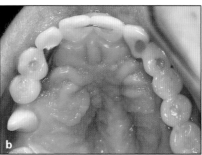

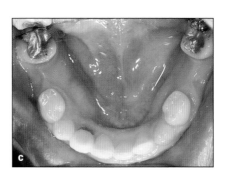

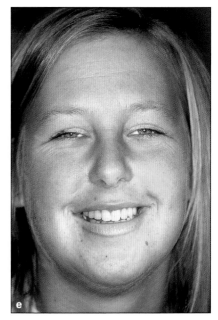

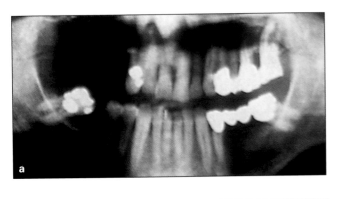
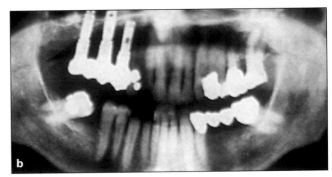
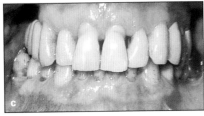
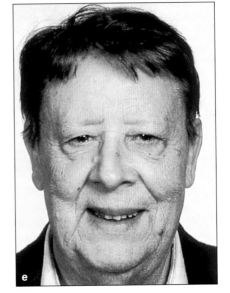
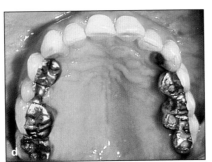

**Fig 2-8** Radiographic *(a and b)*, intraoral *(c and d)*, and frontal *(e)* views of the results of treatment in the posterior maxillary zone in an elderly man.

recorded differences between titanium and other clinically employed materials. Such observations are frequently regarded as being exclusively academic in nature and their clinical significance dubious or even irrelevant. However, the potential risk inherent to the use of any new material must be considered, because its physical and chemical instability may cause adverse sequelae that only long-term outcome studies can determine. An absence of local or systemic toxic effects and a lack of in vitro carcinogenicity and mutagenicity are mandatory.

For example, various ceramic implants made of yttria–partially stabilized zirconia (Y-PSZ) are now commercially available, although no controlled human clinical study regarding clinical osseointegration outcomes is available. These materials have the potential to become an alternative to titanium implants, particularly because their biologic safety as gliding surfaces in orthopedic surgery has been thoroughly investigated. However, orthopedic Y-PSZ implants have been reported to age in a moist environment, and this potential problem must be studied over time.

## Macroscopic implant design

The majority of commercially available implants that claim osseointegration efficacy are cylindrical. Their design may or may not be threaded or tapered. There is now abundant and compelling evidence to support the effectiveness of threaded implants in maintaining a steady state of bone height after the first year of function. Unthreaded implants, on the other hand, have been shown to be frequently associated with a long-term risk of inability to maintain surrounding bone height levels. There is no clinical evidence favoring one thread size type over another, although preliminary evidence suggests that microthreaded implants appear to maintain higher bone levels, at least in the short term. Furthermore, a recent review con-

**Fig 2-9** Laboratory cast *(a)*, and reflected intraoral views *(b and c)* of treatment in the posterior mandibular zone in an elderly woman *(d)*.

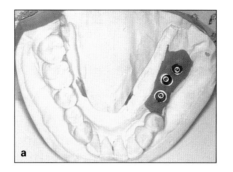
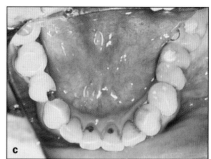
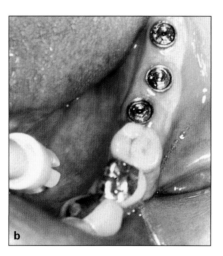
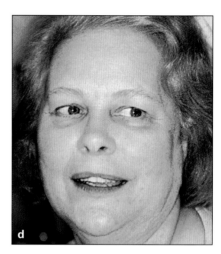

cluded that implant dimensions do not appear to adversely influence treatment outcomes (see chapter 5). Nevertheless, it appears prudent to ensure that a serious discrepancy does not exist between the volume of the cancellous bone at the host site and the volume of the implant.

## Microscopic implant design

An implant's surface is regarded as very important in terms of both its quantitative and qualitative aspects. Quantitative differences refer to surface topography, with roughness being the most frequently exploited property for differentiating commercial initiatives. In fact, moderately rough surfaces have been shown to work better in qualitatively compromised bone. They also appear to have at least equally good results as machined surface implants in favorable host bone sites. This feature has been the most significant design change since the initial introduction of Brånemark's machine-turned commercially pure titanium implant. The premise is that surface roughness increases the potential for rapid bony ingrowths, which in turn permit earlier and even more reliable implant anchorage. In other words, the provision of controllably large volumetric spaces for bone ingrowth should ensure the requisite stability to optimize the interfacial osteogenesis.

However, it is still not known how much bone contact is needed for an implant to be successful or whether different amounts of such contact are required for different host bone sites or for different occlusal loads over time. Furthermore, the range of prepared surface roughness differs and actually elicits different degrees of bone fixation.

Specific topographic characterizations are clearly essential for a reliable interpretation of the precise role of implant surface roughness for bone incorporation. In the absence of this much-needed precise information and an understanding of the contribution of surface roughness to predictable clinical outcomes, the dentist is vulnerable to being misled by commercial promotional concerns rather than scientifically based principles.

The qualitative aspect of an implant's microscopically designed surface refers to the potential for employing bioactive surfaces to influence the nature of the interfacial osteogenesis. Examples include potentially bone-stimulating bioactive surfaces, such as oxidized implants, and surfaces treated with bone-stimulating factors. However, rigorous clinical trials reflecting the long-term beneficial merits of such novel approaches are still unavailable.

## Host site and implant bed

Some patients are clearly not good candidates for osseointegration. Their systemic health may be brittle, they may have undergone irradiation, and their bone may be quantitatively and qualitatively compromised in both local and even generalized edentulous sites. Moreover, they may take medications with the potential for disturbing bone metabolism. They might have also lost their teeth because of periodontal disease, a condition that some authors even regard as a relative contraindication for the osseointegration protocol. Nonetheless, a very large body of clinical research underscores the potential of bone to heal predictably well from a surgically induced wound and anchor the selected alloplastic material that is "screwed into" the planned defect. This phenomenon occurs in heterogeneous population groups, irrespective of age or sex, as long as the host sites are healthy. It has been shown to be influenced by local and systemic health conditions, medications, irradiation, and behavioral habits such as smoking. It certainly appears to be self-evident that a prudent osseointegration protocol demands a healthy host bone site, which must be scrupulously imaged, and a systemic health history that reveals the patient to be in a nonbrittle state.

## Surgical protocols

Current recommendations for the standard optimal surgical approach have changed very little from the originally described protocol. The evolved surgical mantra remains a scrupulously applied one of minimal tissue trauma. The explicit objective is a gentle surgical technique with profuse saline cooling and controlled rotational torque during implant insertion to avoid stress concentrations in adjacent bone.

What has significantly changed, though, has been the expansion of the scope for implant placement. It resulted from an increased understanding of applied surgical principles to deficient bony sites as well as the honing of fine surgical skills, particularly in the context of soft tissue management protocols. While clearly essential to ensure osseointegration, excellent surgical skill is also mandatory because numerous surgical reports have underscored the variable results obtained by different individuals. While the importance of scrupulous surgical protocol is a given, the need for surgical skill must never be overlooked, particularly when less than ideal sites are selected. This is a sobering thought given the nature of training acquired from short continuing education courses that emphasize simulated surgical protocols.

## Loading and prosthodontic protocols

Brånemark's original clinical formula was readily reconciled with the large repertoire of available prosthodontic procedures. These versatile clinical techniques had evolved in response to a need to compensate for different degrees of deficit in a reliable support mechanism. While this proved to be an important treatment planning and application advance, it also led to a desire to speed the process of restoring patients' depleted dentitions. This initiative accelerated even further with the introduction of rough-surface implants and the impressive advances in surgical skills and innovation. The result has been one that offers considerable promise of contracted treatment times and the popularization of altered loading protocols, such as immediate loading in selected cases.

# CLINICAL BENEFITS OF OSSEOINTEGRATION

The demonstrated efficacy and effectiveness of osseointegration, which underscore its suitability for routine clinical application, are summarized in Box 2-2.

## Patient-mediated acceptance

Numerous studies have identified patient expectations and perceptions of what should result from treatment interventions. Patients want:

- To live as long as possible
- To function normally
- To be free of pain or other physical, psychologic, or social symptoms
- To be free of iatrogenic problems from any treatment regimen
- To remain financially solvent after treatment completion

These patient-determined criteria highlight the importance of a biopsychosocial model for disease and health and should arguably underscore all therapeutic interventions. In fact, all of the objectives above can be routinely achieved with applied osseointegration in dental practices, even if quantifiable and universally accepted quality-of-life measures cannot always be employed. While it could be argued that implant-supported prostheses are not in the category of life-prolonging therapy, they are a significant source of enrichment of the patient's quality of life. This is particularly true when the treatment is prescribed to rectify a chronic history of prosthesis maladaptation.

## Stable and retained prostheses

Many patients continue to benefit from wearing removable partial dentures and complete dentures. Yet it is unlikely that all these patients enjoy an uninterrupted sense of security with their dentures. This is compellingly demonstrated by several facts:

- Most denture-wearers will require lifelong servicing of their prostheses to ensure optimal oral health.
- Consumer surveys in different countries reveal that approximately one of every three denture-wearers uses a denture adhesive product in any given year. Denture adhesive sales in North America, for example, are in the range of several million dollars a year.
- Psychologic, esthetic, functional, and social considerations affect patients' perceptions about their denture-wearing experiences.

All of these realities only confirm the profound and insidiously adverse ecologic changes associated with the entire removable prosthesis–wearing experience. Furthermore, no amount of professional skill or improved materials will rectify problems encountered by prosthetically maladaptive patients. The most significant cause of such patient dissatisfaction seems to be lack of prosthetic stability—a constant reminder of the denture's intrusive nature.

Our early studies on the predicament of edentulism confirmed that even an abbreviated form of osseointegration therapy—the overdenture approach—can significantly address the problem. As a result, the attitude of stoic resignation on the part of both patient and dentist that used to be required to address the predicament is now very much a thing of the past.

## Retardation of residual ridge reduction

Time-dependent residual ridge reduction is an irreversible and variable consequence of tooth loss. It may even be accelerated by uncontrollable occlusal functional and parafunctional stresses that cause localized or generalized tissue overload. This compromised and ecologically adverse load-bearing scenario has been shown to be mitigated by provision of endosseous support via implants. Consequently a sustained record of minimally reduced bone height is an integral part of the proposed criteria for determining successful implant treatment outcomes. The quantifiable information about bone behavior around implants has resulted from numerous studies. Detailed and precise measurements of bone height were monitored in heterogeneous patient groups and jawbone sites and in association with different prosthetic designs (Fig 2-10). The accuracy and reliability of the techniques used confirmed the feasibility of a time-dependent

---

**Box 2-2** ROUTINE AND PREDICTABLE CLINICAL YIELDS FROM OSSEOINTEGRATION

- Favorable patient-mediated acceptance
- Stable and retained prostheses
- Retardation of residual ridge reduction
- Minimal risk of morbidity

---

steady state in bone height for the vast majority of the implant abutments. These collective measurements provided important evidence regarding the retardation of residual ridge reduction as opposed to conventional values for such sites under removable prostheses.

The correlation between bone level and long-term implant stability appears to be highly relevant to treatment outcomes. It is clear that a mobile implant is a failure even if it appears to be surrounded by very adequate bone height, because mobility is a reflection of a fibrous rather than a bony interface. Nonetheless, an immobile and painless implant with recorded progressive bone loss suggests a poor prognosis. The precise reasons for bone changes around implants are far from clear. However, the information gleaned from the various studies on bone level behavior around implants over prolonged time frames and in diverse situations should be regarded as integral to the outcome success criteria. We therefore regard long-term painless implant immobility, accompanied by a steady bone state, as indicative of a favorable outcome prognosis. Moreover, this is the sort of information that should be provided by all implant systems so as to better differentiate scientifically tenable treatment outcome claims from commercially defined ones.

## Minimal risk of morbidity

The surgical literature and extensive clinical experience confirm the importance of clinical judgment, meticulous planning, and surgical execution, in addition to scrupulous regard for the importance of postoperative prosthodontic loading, to the routinely achieved successful results. Surgical morbidity is rarely reported and most unlikely to be related to the inherent aspects of the recommended surgical protocols. Furthermore, implants have virtually no adverse ecologic impact on overall oral health. Previous prosthodontic and preprosthetic surgical protocols invariably risked an unpredictable biologic price by

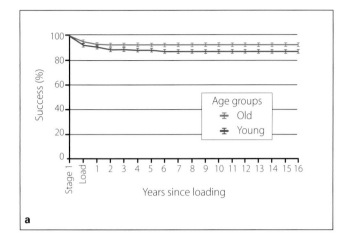

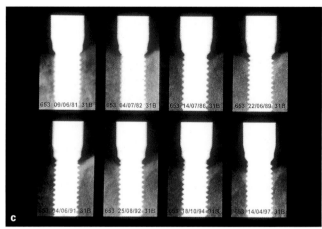

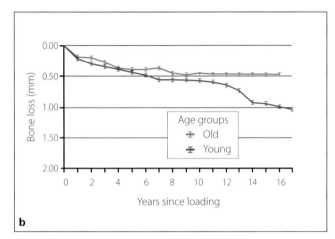

**Fig 2-10** Bryant's documentation of cumulative implant success *(a)* and cumulative mean annual bone loss *(b)* in elderly patients resulted from prospective scrupulous monitoring of bone behavior around loaded implants in matched but different age groups. In *(c)*, bone levels around implants were measured using a reliably repeatable protocol that demonstrated the quantifiable amount of cervical bone change around each implant over a period of several years of study. This methodologic rigor provides irrefutable insights regarding the retardation of ridge resorption around successfully integrated implants.

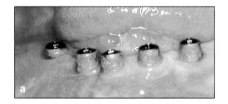

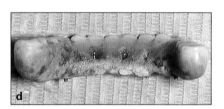

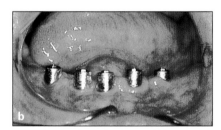

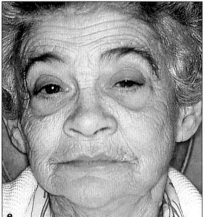

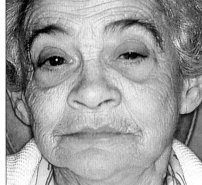

**Fig 2-11** *(a to e)* The inability of this elderly and systemically brittle woman to maintain a program of home care had little impact on her implant-related oral ecology. Photographs were taken during one of her regular follow-up visits several years after her treatment was completed. Clinical experience suggests that less than optimal bone quality, and indeed a history of poor oral hygiene maintenance, may not be compelling deterrents for prescribing osseointegration therapy.

**Box 2-3** DETERMINANTS OF TREATMENT OUTCOME IN IMPLANT PROSTHODONTICS*

The following considerations for successful outcomes with implant-supported prostheses were proposed:

1. Implant therapy is prescribed to resolve prosthodontic problems and permits diverse prosthodontic treatments, which in turn may have an impact on the economics of the service. Such prostheses should meet the clinically evolved standards of function, comfort, and esthetics. They should also allow for routine maintenance and should permit planned or unplanned revisions of the existing design. Criteria of treatment outcome success for implant-supported prostheses should be assessed in the context of time-dependent considerations for any required retreatment.

2. Criteria for implant success apply to individual endosseous implants and include the following:

   • *At the time of testing, the implants have been under functional loading.*

   • *All implants under investigation must be accounted for.*

   • *Because a gold standard for mobility assessment is currently unavailable, the method used must be specifically described in operative terms.*

   • *Radiographs to measure bone loss should be standard periapical films with specified reference points and angulations.*

The success criteria comprise the following determinants:

1. The resultant implant support does not preclude the placement of a planned functional and esthetic prosthesis that is satisfactory to both patient and dentist.

2. No pain, discomfort, altered sensation, or infection is attributable to the implants.

3. Individual unattached implants are immobile when tested clinically.

4. The mean vertical bone loss is less than 0.2 mm annually after the first year of function.

*As discussed at the symposium "Towards Optimized Treatment Outcomes for Dental Implants," held at the University of Toronto, April 24–25, 1998.*

virtue of their inherent intrusiveness and resultant changes in the oral environment.

The practical question of operating in poor quality or osteoporosis-like bone deserves mention. Several experienced surgeons have observed that the main reason for the inferior results reported in poor-quality bone is technique rather than the implant-bone interface. They contend that the initial failure to adequately stabilize an implant is fraught with risk and that the bone's architectural shortcomings frequently can be overcome with a modified surgical approach.

Poor-quality bone does not automatically imply poor healing capacity (Fig 2-11). It can be managed with even more meticulous surgical preparation, a longer healing interval, and delayed loading. Osteoporotic patients demonstrate healing of fractures that is comparable to that among patients without osteoporosis; the process simply takes longer, provided that sufficient initial stability of the traumatized site is present (see chapters 4 and 7).

# SUCCESSFUL OUTCOME CRITERIA

A major reason for the effectiveness of today's implant treatment approach is the result of ongoing efforts by clinical scientists to establish reproducible criteria for clinical success. The premise is that the application of such criteria will enable implant therapy to logically and selectively eclipse traditional prosthodontic replacements in the domains of efficacy and effectiveness.

Albrektsson and colleagues proposed the first criteria for osseointegration success in the 1980s. The proposed determinants were an exclusive outgrowth of the long-term data recorded for the Brånemark system. The standards provided a yardstick, and in many ways a challenge, for other implant systems to provide comparable or even superior data on treatment outcomes. The criteria were fine-tuned slightly over the years and were reviewed at an international symposium in 1998 (Box 2-3).

These criteria are still regarded as less than optimal by a number of clinical researchers because the assessments are partially based on fallible resolution levels (eg, office radiographic imaging) and because they support a dichotomous, all-or-none diagnosis (mobile or immobile; painful or painless; absent or present interfacial radiolucency). Consequently, they do not lend themselves to an entire range of quantifiable success norms.

However, these criticisms tend to ignore the fact that the proposed criteria reflect a synthesis of repeatable recorded observations by numerous colleagues on heterogeneous population groups and in diverse intraoral locales. They have proven to be useful and reliable in the formulation and application of a yardstick to determine success.

Furthermore, most of the commercially available systems still lack long-term studies to establish reliable outcomes for their product. Hence their promotional information is long on claims but short on relevant and plausible data; other systems proposed their own criteria, which were not always of comparable standard, while a few based their outcome data on guidelines that are identical to those presented. The latter approach is a most welcome one since it empowers both dentist and patient to be better informed about their clinical decisions and guarantees an ongoing commitment to the principle of *primum non nocere*—first, do not harm. The alternative has been the risk of a free-for-all commercial culture that could threaten to dominate dental practice. The authors therefore hasten to acknowledge the merits of these criteria and endorse their scope and intentions.

It is clearly unrealistic, and perhaps even naïve, to expect different implant companies to embark on long-term studies comparing the longitudinal merits of one implant over another. However, it is opportune to remember that a 1998 symposium recognized the convergence of clinical certainties that already exist. Common sense, clinical prudence, professional integrity, and scrupulous documentation have already yielded predictable and safe directions for managing abutment loss with implant-supported and -retained prostheses. It seems reasonable to assert that the inherently robust healing potential of human bone remains the major determinant of the induced interfacial osteogenesis or osseointegration and to infer that implant design variations may very well reflect commercial hype that detracts from the authentic issues of judgment, skill, and clinical prudence.

# RECOMMENDED READING

Academy of Osseointegration. State of the Science on Implant Dentistry. [Proceedings of the Consensus Conference on the State of the Science on Implant Dentistry. 3–6 Aug 2006, Oak Brook, IL]. Int J Oral Maxillofac Implants 2007;22(suppl):1–226.

Albrektsson T. Is surgical skill more important for clinical success than changes in implant hardware? Clin Implant Dent Relat Res 2001;3:174–175.

Albrektsson T, Brånemark PI, Hansson HA, Lindstrom J. Osseointegrated titanium implants. Acta Orthop Scand 1981;52,155–170.

Albrektsson T, Wennerberg A. Oral implant surfaces: Part 1—Review focusing on topographic and chemical properties of different surfaces and in vivo response to them. Int J Prosthodont 2004;17:536–543.

Albrektsson T, Wennerberg A. Oral implant surfaces: Part II—Review focusing on clinical knowledge on different surfaces. Int J Prosthodont 2004; 17:536–543.

Albrektsson T, Zarb G, Worthington P, Eriksson RA. The long-term efficacy of currently used dental implants. Int J Oral Maxillofac Implants 1986;1: 11–25.

Bryant SR. The effects of age, jaw site, and bone condition on oral implant outcomes. Int J Prosthodont 1998;11:470–490.

Bryant R, Zarb G. Crestal bone loss proximal to oral implants in older and younger adults. J Prosthet Dent 2003;89:589–597.

European Association for Osseointegration. First EAO Consensus Conference. [Proceedings of the First EAO Consensus Conference, 16–19 Feb 2006, Pfäffikon, Switzerland]. Clin Oral Implants Res 2006;17(suppl 2):1–162.

Lee DW, Choi YS, Park KH, Kim CS, Moon IS. Effect of microthread on the maintenance of marginal bone level: A 3-year prospective study. Clin Oral Implants Res 2007;18:465–470.

Slagter KW, Raghoebar GM, Vissink A. Osteoporosis and edentulous jaws. Int J Prosthodont 2008;21:19–26.

Zarb GA, Albrektsson T. Towards optimized treatment outcomes for dental implants [conference proceedings]. Int J Prosthodont 1998;11:385–521.

Zarb GA, Schmitt A. The longitudinal clinical effectiveness of osseointegrated dental implants: The Toronto Study. J Prosthet Dent 1990;64:53–61.

# 3

# LOCAL AND SYSTEMIC HEALTH CONSIDERATIONS

S. ROSS BRYANT  |  SREENIVAS KOKA  |  IAN R. MATTHEW

Successful implant prosthodontic therapy requires scrupulous attention to local and systemic health concerns. The transition to a scientific era for use of endosseous dental implants saw osseointegration established as a predictable wound-healing phenomenon. The yield has been a satisfying one for both partially and completely edentulous patients seeking stable bone-anchored prostheses with minimal morbidity, despite a diversity of patient-specific risk factors that require attention (Figs 3-1 to 3-3).

Systematic reviews of implant outcome studies suggest that continued high mean rates of survival can be achieved for oral implants, in the range of 80% to 95% success over 10 years or more. Furthermore, mean crestal bone loss around implants is similar to that seen around healthy aging teeth with a long-term average of substantially less than 0.1 mm annually after the first year of function, regardless of arch location or dentate status. Such outcomes align well with other major success criteria for osseointegrated implants: primarily immobility of individual implants, accompanied by a lack of pain and pathology. However, the ability to predict implant failure with specificity and sensitivity, particularly the tendency for implant

or prosthetic failures to cluster in certain patients, has proved elusive. Although most patients experience success of all implants, about 1 or 2 in 10 patients has at least one implant failure, and occasionally multiple implant failures can occur in certain patients, suggesting the need to consider patient-specific characteristics in attempts to predict outcomes.

Achieving the required initial and ongoing stability of the interface between the implant surface and bone has been associated with a balance of factors: selection and design of alloplastic materials; the repertoire of surgical and prosthetic techniques; and treatment planning based on a scrupulous assessment of patient-specific factors that influence the initial and ongoing host bone response. The aim of this chapter is to review common local and systemic health considerations that patients bring to the dental implant equation, including an introduction to site-specific aspects of host bone that are influenced by age, sex, and common systemic conditions or their treatments. Furthermore, common behavioral characteristics that may compromise successful osseointegrated dental implant therapy are discussed.

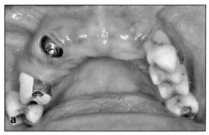
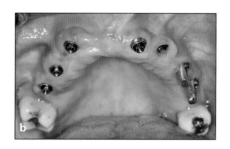
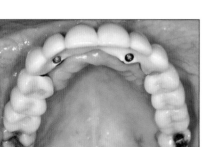
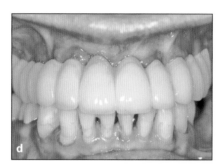
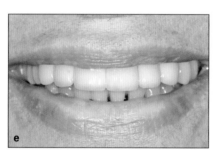

**Fig 3-1** *(a)* A 65-year-old partially edentulous patient with breast cancer history, treated 5 years prior with lumpectomy, radiation, and chemotherapy and currently taking an oral dose of 25 mg exemestane (an aromatase inhibitor to reduce estrogen load) daily. She required extraction of her remaining maxillary premolars and canines because of periodontal disease. Following healing she was managed with three metal-ceramic prostheses on a total of seven threaded titanium implants *(b to e)*, which were placed following careful planning with comprehensive imaging of the proposed sites and autogenous bone grafts placed to optimize bone width in the maxillary anterior and bone height bilaterally in the maxillary sinuses.

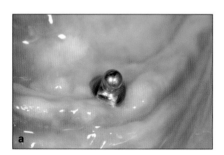
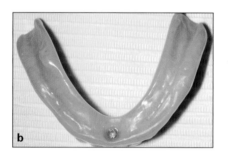
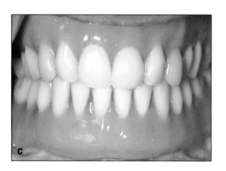
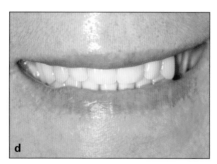

**Fig 3-2** A 70-year-old completely edentulous woman with a 40-year smoking history of a half pack of cigarettes daily in addition to osteoporosis, which had been treated (starting 36 months prior to her implant therapy) with ongoing cycles of 14 days of 400 mg oral etidronate disodium daily (an oral bisphosphonate to increase bone density) followed by 76 days of 1,250 mg of oral calcium carbonate daily. *(a to d)* She was managed with a conventional maxillary complete denture opposing a mandibular overdenture retained by a single threaded titanium implant placed in the midline.

**Fig 3-3** A 79-year-old partially edentulous male patient with evident attrition and self-reported history of bruxism. *(a to e)* He was managed with bilateral posterior fixed implant prostheses (with gold occlusal surfaces) on a total of five threaded titanium implants (one per tooth being replaced), followed by occlusal appliance therapy to help mitigate the risk of occlusal overload at night.

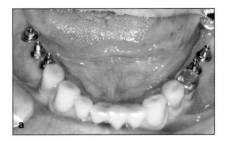
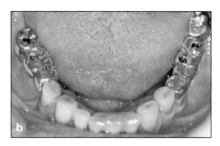
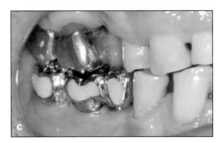
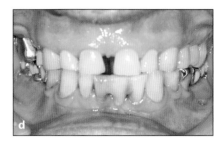
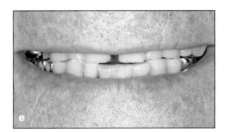

# LOCAL HOST BONE CONSIDERATIONS

## Bone condition and oral implant failure

Bone-anchored prostheses require a sufficient quantity and quality of host bone to stabilize an adequate number of appropriately positioned implants to support prosthetic needs while preserving the integrity of vital structures. Currently there is no generally accepted volume or quality of bone considered necessary and sufficient to house an endosseous implant. However, it is postulated that a bone volume permitting placement of an implant 4 mm in diameter and 10 mm in length is the minimum desirable to promote successful long-term implant-based therapy. Of course, implant design specifications may vary depending on surgical and prosthetic needs as well as requirements for bone and/or soft tissue augmentation procedures.

Bone volume can be diminished by resorption, resection, or deficient development. However, substantial oral bone loss is often a consequence of tooth extraction that culminates in vertical and horizontal resorption of the jaws. Rapid vertical re-

sorption of the residual ridge often occurs during the first year after tooth extraction, slowing thereafter, so that 10 years post-extraction the average rate is only 0.05 mm per year in the edentulous maxilla and 0.20 mm per year in the edentulous mandible. Resorption of the maxilla may leave the ridge crest close to the maxillary sinus or nasal cavity, while posterior mandibular resorption resulting in crestal bone approximating the mandibular canal may preclude implant placement unless bone augmentation is undertaken.

Optimal bone quality is less well understood in the context of dental implant therapy. Indeed, the term *bone quality* itself is prone to variations in interpretation. In this chapter bone quality refers to the structural characteristics of bone that influence the initial formation and subsequent maintenance of an osseointegrated implant-host interface.

Human jawbone quality varies substantially both within and between individuals in characteristics of cortical porosity, cancellous density, the cellular constituents of marrow spaces, and trabecular architecture. Characteristically, the maxillary cortex is thinner than the mandibular cortex. Low-density cancellous bone is typical of the posterior mandible and is also fairly common in the posterior maxilla. Diminished bone quantity and

**Table 3-1   Bone condition and cumulative success rate (CSR) of dental implants**

| Bone | Load period | No. of patients | Overall CSR (No. of implants) | CSR by LZ* bone quantity | CSR by LZ* bone quality |
|---|---|---|---|---|---|
| Edentulous mandible | 4–17 y | 114 | 86% (485) | NS | NS |
| Edentulous maxilla[†] | 4–16 y | 25 | 85% (132) | A, B ≥ 95%[‡] C, D, E ≤ 50%[‡] | 3 = 88%[‡] 4 = 67%[‡] |

*Lekholm and Zarb (LZ) classification: bone quantity, types A to E; bone quality, types 1 to 4.
[†]Maxillary type 1 and 2 jaws were not treated.
[‡]Difference between groups is statistically significant (Wilcoxon P < .05).
NS = differences across groups are not statistically significant.

**Table 3-2   Effects of bone condition and years of edentulism on mean crestal bone loss (CBL) for dental implants after first year of load**

| Bone | Load period | No. of prosthetic sites | CBL after 1st y (No. of implants) | CBL by LZ* bone quantity | CBL by LZ* bone quality | CBL by years of edentulism at implant placement |
|---|---|---|---|---|---|---|
| Pooled maxillary/ mandibular sites | 4–17 y | 98 | 0.04 mm/y (385) | A = 0.05 mm/y[†] B = 0.08 mm/y[†] C = 0.02 mm/y[†] D = 0.002 mm/y[†] E = 0.03 mm/y[†] | NS | ≤ 1 y = 0.11 mm/y[†] 2 to 4 y = 0.09 mm/y[†] 5 to 9 y = 0.04 mm/y[†] 10 to 24 y = 0.03 mm/y[†] ≥ 25 y = 0.01 mm/y[†] |

*Lekholm and Zarb (LZ) classification: bone quantity, types A to E; bone quality, types 1 to 4.
[†]Difference between groups is statistically significant (ANOVA P < .01).
NS = differences across groups are not statistically significant.

poor bone quality, as measured radiographically according to the Lekholm and Zarb (LZ) classification (see Fig 1-16), have been associated with reduced short-term success of dental implants. However, when the complex physiology of bone as a tissue is combined with the nuances of the variable response of each host osteotomy site, no single classification system is able to describe all of the pertinent parameters of bone quality. This limitation may be remedied in the future as better imaging measures of bone quality become available and correlations to implant survival or success are determined.

Clinical evidence of up to 17 years follow-up at the University of Toronto (Table 3-1) shows that overall success of machined titanium implants placed in the anterior segment of more than 100 consecutively treated edentulous mandibles was not significantly different across the range of LZ bone quantity or quality categories. In contrast, the success of machined titanium implants in 25 consecutively treated edentulous maxillae did vary statistically by bone condition. The cumulative success rate was only 67% among maxillary implants in low-density cancellous bone (LZ type 4) and only 50% or

less among implants in more resorbed maxillae (LZ type C, D, or E) where only basal bone remained. However, the statistical significance of bone quantity and quality was inconsistent in multivariate modeling when various independently significant variables were assessed concurrently—likely in part because relatively few resorbed maxillae were treated in this study or as a result of the vagaries of the concept of bone quality.

## Bone condition and crestal bone loss

In view of the tendency for the rate of resorption of edentulous jaws to be greatest immediately following extraction, the question arises whether the rate of crestal bone loss is greater around implants placed in recent extraction sites, particularly those in less resorbed jaws. Results of attempts to examine this supposition have been inconclusive in the short term. Long-term (10-year) evidence has demonstrated that less preoperative resorption and shorter preoperative periods of edentulism could predict part of an elevated tendency for crestal bone resorption

| TABLE 3-3 | IMPACT OF COMMON BEHAVIORAL AND SYSTEMIC FACTORS ON ORAL IMPLANT FAILURE | |
| --- | --- | --- |
| Risk | Behavioral | Systemic |
| Low | Correct oral hygiene | Age* and sex* <br> Systemic osteoporosis <br> Controlled cardiovascular disease <br> Controlled hypothyroidism <br> Controlled diabetes mellitus* <br> History of periodontitis* |
| Possible increase | Parafunction | Hormone replacement therapy* <br> Oral bisphosphonate therapy* <br> Corticosteroid therapy* <br> Sjögren syndrome <br> Vitamin D–dependent rickets <br> Active chemotherapy |
| Known increase | Cigarette smoking | Irradiation |

*Some conflicting evidence exists.

observed surrounding machined titanium implants in such sites. Reinforcing this finding was the University of Toronto study described previously that demonstrated a statistically, but unlikely to be clinically, significant tendency for slightly less than average crestal bone loss, 0.03 mm or less annually after the first year, among machined titanium implants placed in groups with the most resorbed jaws (LZ types C, D, and E) compared to 0.05 mm or more annually after the first year among implants placed in groups with less resorbed jaws (LZ type A or B) (Table 3-2). However, neither jawbone quantity nor quality could fully explain the variation in crestal bone loss when multivariate statistical modeling was employed. In general, regardless of the time interval between implant placement and prior tooth extraction, slower crestal bone loss appears to occur when compared with that experienced by bone that does not house a dental implant.

# BEHAVIORAL AND SYSTEMIC HEALTH CONSIDERATIONS

Increasing efforts have been made in recent years to document the possible impact of several patient-related systemic and behavioral factors that could act to impair the bone-healing and remodeling response required for dental implants. In addition to age and sex, these factors comprise common systemic conditions or their treatments, for example, osteoporosis, diabetes

mellitus, irradiation, cardiovascular diseases, hypothyroidism, and periodontal diseases, and common behavioral characteristics, such as oral hygiene impairment, smoking, and parafunction. Among them, smoking, diabetes mellitus, and irradiation have perhaps received the most research attention (Table 3-3). However, since several of these conditions often coexist and cannot be ethically manipulated for randomized controlled trial assignments, studies to distinguish their individual contributions have proven difficult and in some cases have provided contradictory findings.

## Age and sex

Consistent with the rest of the skeleton, the human jaws tend to suffer increased cortical porosity and impaired cancellous density and architecture with aging. Advanced age increases the risk for systemic illnesses, such as osteoporosis, that can negatively affect bone physiology. The frailty of old age may also diminish oral hygiene efforts, leading to increased local irritants around dental implants. Fortunately, studies continue to indicate that oral implant outcomes are comparable among older and younger adults, suggesting that old age itself will not influence the potential for sustaining stable oral implants. Likewise, although growing children and adolescents appear to have normal potential for osseointegration, the preponderance of evidence suggests that caution should be exercised in planning dental implants for growing individuals because of the relatively unpredictable consequences of continued jaw growth and

**TABLE 3-4   CUMULATIVE SUCCESS RATE (CSR) OF IMPLANTS, BY AGE GROUPS**

| Study | Load period | Older patients | | Younger patients | |
|---|---|---|---|---|---|
| | | Age range (No. of patients) | CSR (No. of implants) | Age range (No. of patients) | CSR (No. of implants) |
| Bryant and Zarb* | 4–16 y | 66–74 y (39) | 92% NS (190) | 26–49 y (43) | 87% NS (184) |
| Engfors et al[†] | 5 y | 80–93 y (133) | Max = 93% NS (282); Mand = 99.5% NS (479) | 41–79 y (115) | Max = 93% NS (336); Mand = 99.7% NS (334) |

*Partially and completely edentulous, maxillary and mandibular sites.
[†]Completely edentulous, maxillary (max) and mandibular (mand) sites.
NS = differences between age groups are not statistically significant (Wilcoxon P < .05).

development on jaw relationships and implant position. Regardless, if implants are placed in young patients, regular prosthetic revisions may be anticipated until growth is completed.

Two studies comparing older and younger adult groups for follow-up periods of at least 4 years confirmed that no statistical differences in implant success should be expected in relation to age (Table 3-4); in both studies, machined titanium implants were used. The earlier study found no significant differences in either cumulative implant success or the rates of crestal bone loss over 4 to 16 years of function, despite the fact that the older group had more physical frailties and systemic illness. To reduce extraneous influences, the patients were matched closely, making them identical or very similar on the basis of sex, implant number and location, prosthetic plan, condition of the opposing dentition, and year of implant placement. Mean annual crestal bone loss observed around the implants in the edentulous jaws in both groups was less than 0.05 mm per year after the first year of loading.

Likewise, a more recent study also found no significant difference in either cumulative implant success or mean rates of crestal bone loss over 5 years of function, in this case comparing consecutively treated older and younger edentulous adults with fixed implant prostheses. Slightly more than two-thirds of the older group had mandibular prostheses, compared to slightly less than two-thirds of the younger group. The mean annual crestal bone loss observed around the implants in the edentulous arches in both groups was 0.05 mm per year or less after the first year of loading.

## Osteoporosis

Controlled prospective studies of the impact of systemic osteoporosis on oral implant failure have yet to be conducted. It is known that skeletal bone loss is more common in aging women, particularly postmenopausal women, than men, ostensibly reflecting a reduction in sex hormone levels that predisposes the individual to systemic osteoporosis. This condition appears to result from increased bone remodeling, whereby bone resorption slightly exceeds formation, particularly in cancellous bone. This site-specific nature could partly explain why the most serious manifestation of osteoporosis, bone fracture, typically manifests as fractures of the vertebrae (spine), the wrist, or the proximal femur (hip).

It has been difficult to establish a link between systemic osteoporosis and oral bone loss. Perhaps not surprisingly then, preliminary studies in animals and humans suggest that systemic osteoporosis is not associated with diminished success of osseointegration. A systematic review of the relationship between osseointegration and systemic disease found very high overall implant survival rates reported in small retrospective case series on the outcome of dental implants in patients with systemic osteoporosis. The longest reported study found success rates of at least 97% for both maxillary and mandibular implants over 6 months to 11 years in 16 women diagnosed with systemic osteoporosis. Data published after the aforementioned systematic review clearly show, in a relatively large subject population (almost 200 subjects) followed for up to 10 years (mean approximately 4.5 years), that a diagnosis of osteoporosis or osteopenia in postmenopausal women with known bone mineral density scores does not affect implant survival rates compared with survival rates in postmenopausal women with a normal bone mineral density score using the World Health Organization (WHO) classification system. These data strongly support the notion that a diagnosis of systemic osteoporosis is not a contraindication for implant placement.

The use of exogenous corticosteroids may also induce a reduction of bone density—secondary osteoporosis—and consequently pose an increased risk for dental implant failure. However, to date there are few reports investigating the effect of corticosteroid therapy on implant survival and success, and those available suggest dental implants can be successful in patients receiving corticosteroid therapy.

## Oral bisphosphonates

Recent attention has highlighted clinical concern that bisphosphonate drug therapy may predispose patients to osteonecrosis of the jaws (ONJ), a condition whereby osseous healing is compromised, leaving exposed bone uncovered by mucosa for longer than 6 to 8 weeks. In some cases, enduring bone exposure, chronic pain, and even substantial bone loss predisposing to pathologic fracture of the jawbones may ensue.

Bisphosphonates are powerful drug mediators of bone remodeling used presently in oral forms often for the prevention and treatment of bone loss associated with systemic osteoporosis. The therapeutic goal is to mitigate the serious risks of morbidity and mortality associated with fracture of the spine, wrist, or hip. Bisphosphonates are also used intravenously in significantly higher doses to manage bone resorption in cancer patients with bone metastasis and to diminish the associated risk of skeletal events, including osteolysis, fracture, and bone pain.

The incidence of and risk factors for bisphosphonate-associated ONJ are not yet precisely known. In one study of patients taking oral bisphosphonate, the risk of ONJ was estimated at less than 4 in 1 million users, suggesting that the condition may either be idiopathic or occur in the presence of one or more cofactors. However, another study cites the risk of ONJ in those who take oral bisphosphonates and who have had a recent dental extraction as 1 in 296. Clearly, the field is in great need of further data to establish the true risk and incidence of ONJ in osteoporosis-directed bisphosphonate users. The main dental factors that appear to contribute to ONJ are invasive surgery or soft tissue trauma that exposes jawbone. Fortunately, those patients who are likely to need a dental extraction or other form of invasive oral surgery are at low risk of developing ONJ. Overall, the incidence of bisphosphonate-associated ONJ appears to be very low and by far the vast majority of confirmed cases have been in cancer patients taking high-dose intravenous bisphosphonates. The risk may also depend to some extent on the formulation and duration of the drug used.

Very few studies are available pertaining to dental implant use and oral bisphosphonates. A clinical trial of oral implants placed in patients with and without oral bisphosphonates found rates of implant success greater than 99% in both groups over at least 3 years of follow-up and no ONJ in either group. The study involved 210 implants placed in 50 consecutive patients, 25 of whom received a common oral bisphosphonate and 25 age-matched controls who received no bisphosphonate. However, since none of the subjects had previously used bisphosphonates at the start of the trial, the effect of long-term oral bisphosphonate use is unknown.

Maxillary and mandibular bone remodels at a higher rate than most other bones, and hence it takes up oral bisphosphonates at a greater pace, resulting in a relatively high concentration of drug. Given the long half-life for oral bisphosphonates, research documenting the effect of long-term bisphosphonate use on dental implant survival/success is needed.

## Diabetes mellitus

Diabetes mellitus is an increasingly prevalent endocrine disorder associated with impaired circulation and healing and increased susceptibility to infection. Nearly 9 of 10 diabetic patients have the type 2 form of the condition that can routinely be managed with diet, exercise, and oral drugs. The less common form, type 1, requires insulin supplementation to manage blood glucose levels.

In general, diabetic patients have increased risks for oral problems and, as a result, diabetes has been investigated as a risk factor for dental implant failure. A recent systematic review of implant outcomes associated with diabetes found no evidence of implant survival differences when comparing diabetic and nondiabetic patients in several retrospective studies. The pooled estimate of implant survival was 92% for diabetic patients.

In addition, the only study that has compared outcomes in diabetic patients (15 subjects) with matched controls (30 subjects) found no significant difference in risk of implant failure. The diabetic patients were well controlled medically. The results demonstrated just under 7% failure for both groups over a period up to 17 years, and the overall rate of bone loss did not differ between the groups. Thus, controlled diabetes does not in itself appear to be a risk factor for implant failure.

## Irradiation

Although not as common as other age-related diseases, orofacial neoplasms often require management using a combination of resection and irradiation followed by efforts at prosthetic rehabilitation. The stability of maxillofacial prostheses can sometimes be supplemented with osseointegrated implants. However, irradiation therapy increases the risk of osteoradionecrosis and can compromise bone physiology. Therapeutic doses of irradiation are thought to compromise bone physiology by killing osteocytes in the pathway of the beam; by compromising the regenerative potential of periosteum by reducing cellularity, vascularity, and the potential for osteoid formation; and by compromising the patency of blood vessels.

Regardless of the mechanism, an increased risk of implant failure has been associated with irradiation therapy involving greater than 55 Gy, particularly in the maxilla, where cancellous bone density also tends to be lowest. Mucositis is also a common response to irradiation therapy, and this has led to increased risks of soft tissue complications, particularly during the healing phase associated with endosseous implants. Although conclusive data are not available, hyperbaric oxygen has been suggested to improve the success rates of oral implants in irradiated bone, particularly in the maxilla.

## Patient psychology

An impressive arsenal of data exists to measure the technical success of engineering ingenuity involved in osseointegration-based oral therapy. Long-term evidence supports an excellent track record for machined titanium dental implants, and other more recently introduced implant surfaces may ultimately afford similar results. The literature is relatively sparsely populated, however, with psychologic assessments of implant patients and how well osseointegration-based therapy resolves the needs and demands of patients.

Clearly, each patient should be informed of the variety of treatment options to address his or her unique presentation with partial or complete edentulism. These options may or may not include osseointegration as a tool to restore comfort, function, and esthetics. Each of these three factors will be viewed with different degrees of importance by each patient, and the onus is on the practitioner to help the patient choose the form of treatment that best meets his or her needs and desires.

The relative lack of evidence supporting the notion that edentulism leads to significant systemic consequences indicates that replacement of missing teeth does not necessarily improve physical health. It is quite likely that psychosocial factors drive patient demand for replacement of missing teeth. In essence, society's emphasis on appearance may be the most influential circumstance that compels patients to present for a discussion of prosthodontic treatment options. Narby and coworkers have eloquently described some of the interplay between patient demands and patient needs and contend that ideally a careful appraisal of these two factors is warranted.

Ultimately, patient satisfaction is the underpinning of patient-centered care. Patient satisfaction after therapy is most often measured using quality-of-life questionnaires. Results of studies such as these show that, in general, patients treated with osseointegration-based therapy perceive an overall improvement in their oral status (comfort, function, and esthetics) and consequently are satisfied with treatment. However, these re-sults should be interpreted with caution because, occasionally, there are patients who describe an improvement in all of three categories and yet state a high level of dissatisfaction with the outcome. Furthermore, there is evidence that, regardless of the specific prosthodontic treatment provided, edentulous patients with adaptive psychologic capabilities (both physical and psychologic) will feel satisfied with their treatment.

In contrast, there are certain patients who may tend psychologically to be dissatisfied with any form of prosthodontic therapy, even when the practitioner provides the best possible technical result and the patient has endured extensive surgical or other irreversible interventions and financial outlay. In ideal circumstances, patients who will be challenging to satisfy are identified before irreversible therapy of any kind is initiated. There is no accepted and validated mechanism to identify these patients, and it is left to the clinician's intuition to assess the suitability of progressing with treatment; this is a tenuous situation, because it may be that patient personality is the key variable in whether patient satisfaction is attainable.

Clearly, prudent management of patient expectations at the treatment planning stage is a crucial ingredient in creating a recipe for "successful" treatment. Engaging patients in a sincere discussion of their needs, wants, and dental history is imperative to identify the psychologically maladaptive patient, because regret and remorse on behalf of the patient and the practitioner can be the consequences of treating this type of patient.

## Other systemic conditions

In recent years, preliminary evidence on implant outcomes has also been reported for several other systemic conditions that have the potential to impair osseous healing and remodeling and thereby compromise dental implant success. Studies, primarily with small patient samples, have indicated that some increased risk of implant failure may exist in patients with Sjögren syndrome, those with vitamin D–dependent rickets, and in those actively receiving chemotherapy for cancer. Preliminary studies, some with very small numbers, have also indicated no elevation in implant failures among patients with controlled cardiovascular diseases and controlled hypothyroidism, human immunodeficiency virus, acquired immunodeficiency syndrome, hypophosphatasia, scleroderma, Erdheim-Chester disease, and hereditary ectodermal dysplasia.

## Oral hygiene and periodontal disease

Plaque accumulation can be associated with peri-implant mucositis, as is expected when bacteria are allowed to accumulate in contact with mucosa. However, unlike the established rela-

TABLE 3-5 IMPLANT SURVIVAL AMONG CIGARETTE SMOKERS AND NONSMOKERS

| Study | Load period | Implant survival | |
|---|---|---|---|
| | | Smoker | Nonsmoker |
| Klokkevold and Han* | 1–12 y | 89.7%[†] | 93.3%[†] |
| DeLuca and Zarb[‡] | 1–20 y | 76.9%[§] | 86.7%[§] |

*Pooled implant survival based on 14 studies, 1993–2005; 2,394 implants placed in smokers; 5,402 implants placed in nonsmokers.

[†]Difference between groups is statistically significant (Z test P < .01).

[‡]Implant survival by patient, based on crude proportion of patients with failures; 494 implants placed in 104 smokers; 1,045 implants placed in 285 nonsmokers.

[§]Difference between groups is statistically significant (Kaplan-Meier survival analysis P ≤ .01).

tionship between dental plaque and periodontal disease in a relatively small proportion of susceptible individuals, evidence suggests that plaque accumulation per se is a precursor neither of peri-implant bone loss nor of implant failure, at least with machined titanium implants.

Intraoral materials with increased roughness of the surface appear susceptible to accumulating increased quantities of plaque and a shift toward more pathogenic bacteria in the biofilm and resulting inflammation in adjacent mucosa. This suggests the possibility that increased roughness of implant surfaces may contribute to peri-implant inflammation in cases where the rough surface is exposed to plaque. However, the presence or absence of peri-implant soft tissue inflammation is not a predictor of crestal bone loss, as evidenced by a large number of publications describing long-term results in human populations. Unfortunately, despite the preponderance of human evidence invalidating a link between peri-implant soft tissue inflammation and crestal bone loss, some clinician scientists continue to utilize animal models to investigate this flawed assumption.

Recent systematic reviews of studies with up to 10 years of follow-up have confirmed no mean difference in implant survival between patients without periodontitis and patients treated for periodontitis. Pooled implant survival exceeded 95% in both groups. There was no difference in implant failure in patients with and without histories of periodontitis-associated tooth loss, and pooled implant failure rates were less than 8% in both groups. However, measures of success (based primarily on adding soft tissue parameters) did differ between the groups, suggesting that there was more mucosal inflammation in patients with a history of periodontitis.

One 5-year study also noted a statistically significant difference of 0.5 mm greater mean total crestal bone loss around the implants from the time of abutment placement among the periodontitis patients. Based on this finding, the annual rate of bone loss after the first year of loading must have been less than 0.1 mm annually for both groups, so the clinical impact of the purportedly statistically significant difference is inconsequential. The authors of these systematic reviews also acknowledged the difficulty in distinguishing the effect of combined risk factors. For example, it was noted that smoking and periodontal disease may often coexist to such a degree that it would be difficult to distinguish the effects of smoking from those of periodontitis.

## Smoking

Cigarette smoking is known to impair wound healing, and so it also has been studied as a possible risk factor for dental implant failure, both during the initial healing and once osseointegration has been established. Several preliminary studies have suggested that the risk of implant failure is modestly higher among smokers. Furthermore, one study demonstrated that the detrimental effect on implant healing among smokers may be eliminated with their successful participation in a smoking cessation program prior to implant placement surgery. A recent systematic review of implant outcomes associated with smoking confirmed that implant survival (clinically present) and success (immobile with minimal bone loss) were statistically better among nonsmokers than among smokers (Table 3-5). The meta-analysis found a pooled estimate of implant survival among nonsmokers of 93%, a result 3% better than that for smokers in studies ranging from 1 to 12 years. In comparison, the pooled estimate of implant success (based primarily on accounting for crestal bone loss) in the same review was 91% for nonsmokers; this rate was 11% better than that found for smokers, suggesting that some implants in smokers had higher rates of crestal bone loss despite remaining in function.

A more recent pair of studies reinforced and added to these findings over an even longer period of follow-up—up to 20 years. Again, overall failure rates for oral implants were significantly higher for active smokers (see Table 3-5). Furthermore, smoking at the time of implant surgery was associated with a 1.7-times higher incidence of early implant failure (failure before loading), and the risk appeared to be related directly to the quantity of cigarettes smoked. In contrast, late implant failure (failure after loading) was not associated with smoking at the time of implant surgery but was associated with a greater than 25 cigarette-year history (calculated by multiplying the number of years smoked by the typical number of cigarettes used daily). Patients with a positive smoking history had a 1.9-times higher rate of late implant failure than did patients who had never smoked or did not have a greater than 25 cigarette-year history.

Furthermore, the mean rate of crestal bone loss observed in the individuals with a positive smoking history was 0.07 mm annually after the first year of loading compared to 0.04 mm per year among nonsmokers. As with the systematic reviews on periodontitis, the results indicated that the annual rate of bone loss after the first year of loading was less than 0.1 mm annually for both smoking and nonsmoking groups.

In summary, although some practitioners believe that smokers should not receive dental implant therapy, the effect of smoking may be less than previously believed. Smokers should be informed that their risk of implant failure is indeed higher than that among nonsmokers. However, smokers still enjoy relatively high survival rates based on data from 1 to 20 years of follow-up.

## Parafunction

Clenching and bruxism are two of the most difficult forms of oral parafunction to mitigate when planning dental implant therapy. The clinical challenge is to reconcile the subconscious and excessive frequency, duration, and/or magnitude of occlusal contacts with the biologic and technical durability of the implant prosthesis. In the absence of parafunction, masticatory loads are in the region of 20 kg spread over the natural occlusion and generally less with removable dentures, although average loads can recover if implants are used to stabilize the prosthesis. It is also known that functional occlusal contact forces tend to be exerted over less than 20 minutes per day for chewing and swallowing activities, including both daytime and nighttime periods. Maximum biting force can consciously increase masticatory loads up to 5 times in some individuals, and loads up to 20 times the average have been measured.

Excessive forces can also be generated subconsciously during clenching or bruxing over much longer periods and with much greater frequency than functional loading patterns, particularly during sleep. The impact of these forms of parafunction on dental implants and the prostheses they support has yet to be quantified in a valid manner. The difficulty arises at least in part because of deficiencies in either the validity or clinical practicality of measuring parafunction. For example, poorly validated surrogate measures such as patient self-report or tooth wear patterns, along with better validated but less practical direct measures of jaw activity using polysomnography in a sleep laboratory, present the clinician with the challenge of interpretation.

Qualitatively, parafunctional habits have been attributed to oral implant failure both during initial healing and following insertion of the prosthesis. Consequently, immediate and early loading of dental implants has been discouraged in all but optimal conditions, especially when other detrimental factors are present, such as poor primary stability of the implant, that may deter the desired wound-healing response. Higher rates of crestal bone loss and fractures of implants, implant components, or other prosthetic materials have also been complications attributed to parafunctional occlusal forces. However, controlled prospective studies that diagnose patients with parafunction using validated measures to prevent risk-ridden treatment are unavailable for scrutiny.

What remains for the moment is the concept of a therapeutic occlusion that encompasses bilateral occlusal contacts at a comfortable vertical dimension, freedom in the retruded contact position, support distributed around the arch, and forces directed down the long axis of the implants. Even this "optimal" occlusion may not be sufficient to counteract excessive parafunctional forces that overload the host-implant interface or the prosthetic system. In some patients, the consequences of occlusal parafunction may be lessened by an oral occlusal appliance used during peak parafunctional periods such as sleep-associated bruxism.

# Conclusion

Compelling evidence exists that osseointegrated oral implant–based therapy, used in a diversity of age- and site-specific prosthodontic applications, yields predictable, long-term successful treatment outcomes. Based on major criteria for clinically successful osseointegration, oral implants are medically contraindicated primarily in patients whose health is considered sufficiently brittle to preclude any elective surgery. Essentially, a rigorous application of established surgical and prosthodontic protocols will routinely meet with predictable outcomes if the patient is able to undergo minor oral surgery.

However, circumspection is still warranted because there is a lack of evidence describing the extent to which various systemic and behavioral conditions may impose contraindications for oral implant therapy. Ethical constraints preclude randomization of such conditions in a classic experimental sense, and many of these conditions can exist concurrently, making comparative studies fraught with difficulties in distinguishing the various potential effects. Furthermore, data do not exist on the impact of severe conditions simply because the necessary studies have not been conducted.

Inability on the part of a patient to consent to and comply with a necessary range of treatment recommendations is generally a contraindication for treatment. Consequently it is typical to exclude from dental implant therapy those patients with psychoses or other conditions in which informed consent cannot be obtained or who have unrealistic treatment expectations. In addition, patients who are unable or unwilling to manage active oral disease or a nonphysiologic occlusion may not be good candidates for osseointegration-based therapy.

Unfavorable bone quantity and quality, particularly the atrophic maxilla, have been variably associated with implant failure risk. Furthermore, implants placed in sites with shorter periods of edentulism have been associated with elevated crestal bone loss, a finding that may have particular implications for younger adults. The osseointegration of oral implants otherwise appears to be equally successful in older and younger adults with various completely and partially edentulous situations. Preliminary evidence suggests that, if systemic health conditions are stable, oral implant success may not be affected by the common illnesses associated with aging, including cardiovascular diseases, osteoporosis, hypothyroidism, and diabetes mellitus.

Remaining unclear is the effect of diverse patient-mediated concerns as they impact the biologic and psychosocial needs of patients, including those relating to economic outcomes of various prosthodontic treatment strategies. Such assessments are necessary if both the dentist and patient are to collaborate to make the best informed prosthodontic treatment decision, whether or not it includes the use of osseointegrated dental implants.

# Recommended Reading

Bryant SR. The effects of age, jaw site, and bone condition on oral implant outcomes. Int J Prosthodont 1998;11:470–490.

Bryant SR, Zarb GA. Crestal bone loss proximal to oral implants in older and younger adults. J Prosthet Dent 2003;89:589–597.

DeLuca S, Zarb GA. The effect of smoking on osseointegrated dental implants. 2. Peri-implant bone loss. Int J Prosthodont 2006;19:560–566.

Elsubeihi ES, Zarb GA. Implant prosthodontics in medically challenged patients: The University of Toronto experience. J Can Dent Assoc 2002;68: 103–108.

Engfors I, Ortorp A, Jemt T. Fixed implant-supported prostheses in elderly patients: A 5-year retrospective study of 133 edentulous patients older than 79 years. Clin Implant Dent Relat Res 2004;16:190–198.

Esposito M, Hirsch JM, Lekholm U, Thomsen P. Biological factors contributing to failures of osseointegrated oral implants. 2. Etiopathogenesis. Eur J Oral Sci 1998;106:721–764.

Jeffcoat, MJ. Safety of oral bisphosphonates: Controlled studies on alveolar bone. Int J Oral Maxillofac Implants 2006;21:349–353.

Klokkevold PR, Han TJ. How do smoking, diabetes, and periodontitis affect outcomes of implant treatment? Int J Oral Maxillofac Implants 2007; 22(suppl):173–198.

Koka S, Clarke BL, Amin S, Gertz M, Ruggiero SL. Oral bisphosphonate therapy and osteonecrosis of the jaw: What to tell the concerned patient. Int J Prosthodont 2007;20:115–122.

Mombelli A, Cionca N. Systemic diseases affecting osseointegration therapy. Clin Oral Implants Res 2006;17(suppl 2):97–103.

Narby B, Kronström M, Söderfelt B, Palmqvist S. Prosthodontics and the patient. 2. Need becoming demand, demand becoming utilization. Int J Prosthodont 2007;20:183–189.

Schou S, Holmstrup P, Worthington HV, Esposito M. Outcome of implant therapy in patients with previous tooth loss due to periodontitis. Clin Oral Implants Res 2006;17(suppl 2):104–123.

Sennerby L, Roos J. Surgical determinants of clinical success of osseointegrated oral implants: A review of the literature. Int J Prosthodont 1998; 11:408–420.

# 4

# HEALING RESPONSE

TOMAS ALBREKTSSON | VICTORIA FRANKE-STENPORT | ANN WENNERBERG

Preparation of the host site and subsequent placement of an implant lead to a series of healing events and the ultimate response of osseointegration with the alloplastic material prescribed. The process of osseointegration is, however, easily disturbed. Events that can disrupt the process include traumatic surgery that kills nearby cells, the use of unsuitable implant materials, or alterations to the established implant protocol that create biologic challenges and jeopardize the healing response. This chapter will discuss relevant biologic factors that impact the interfacial bone healing response and influence the desired osseointegration.

## BIOLOGIC BACKGROUND TO HOST SITE PREPARATION

Drilling in bone will inevitably result in tissue trauma that will trigger the subsequent healing response. The tissue trauma will sensitize nearby mesenchymal cells, endothelial cells, and to some extent preexisting cells of the bone lineage, while it simultaneously stimulates the release of various types of growth factors. In fact, a maximal healing response is started by a minimal level of surgical trauma since more trauma will definitely not produce a better tissue response but rather will hinder healing by necrotizing cells needed for tissue repair.

It is generally agreed that the major portion of cells that will repair the bone wound are undifferentiated at the time of injury; hence bone healing is dependent on proper guidance of a satisfactory number of these primitive cells to undergo osteogenic induction. However, the early tissue healing response is quite primitive, and a number of different cellular types will be stimulated simultaneously, with the human genetic code determining that a sufficient amount of bone, soft tissues, and blood vessels will be formed—an easily disturbed process.

One such potential disturbance is undue formation of soft fibrous tissue, which is formed more rapidly than bone tissue. There is a risk that such a response will fill the defect before onset of bone formation, an adverse response that may be inhibited by the use of barrier membranes in certain clinical situations.

Another potential problem that may disturb bone healing is movement. Extensive movement permits primitive mesenchymal cells to develop into cells of the soft tissue lineage, and bone healing will be disturbed or even prevented. This potential problem may be clinically controlled by avoiding direct loading, particularly if the implant is placed in vulnerable, poor-quality bone. Movement will then be minimal, and bone healing may ensue in a more predictable manner.

Considerable interest has been focused on potential enhancement of the bone response. One approach has been external administration of growth factors, which are theoretically one way to reinforce the bone response. However, the circumstances in which such outside reinforcement of the bone response is needed remain somewhat unclear.

For the majority of all placed oral implants, the patient's inherent growth factors are sufficient for eliciting a proper healing response, and it remains most uncertain if external administration of more growth factors is of any benefit at all. Nevertheless, it is possible that implants placed in compromised bone beds, or implants that are initially unstable for whatever reason, may actually acquire better bone support if growth factors are administered externally. Therefore, a short overview of growth factors is included in this chapter.

The most essential clinical information related to bone healing—whether about fracture repair or oral implant integration—remains an outgrowth of empirical knowledge. Clinical experience of the trial-and-error variety suggests that certain fractures may require prolonged immobilization (sometimes up to 9 months) for proper bone healing to occur. In contrast, certain other fractures, such as humeral and mandibular ones, may not need any external immobilization at all.

In the case of an oral implant, a conservative, empirically based, but equally valid protocol is to avoid direct loading. This is traditionally achieved via a two-stage surgical procedure with loading of anterior mandibular implants after 3 months, while the posterior mandibular zones and the maxilla are usually assigned a longer healing period of approximately 6 months.

Oral surgical expertise has also borrowed from the orthopedic experience, where certain cases of fracture healing are regarded as not needing immobilization. Consequently, specific implant situations appear to lend themselves to being loaded earlier and perhaps even immediately (same day of placement), provided that their initial stability is satisfactory.

In an ideal situation, neither the surgical insertion nor the subsequent loading of the implant should disturb the healing response. Furthermore, substantial amounts of research have now focused on altering the physical characteristics of implants in an attempt to promote a predictably stronger bone response. Implant design innovations, together with enhanced surgical skills and techniques, have expanded indications for implant placement and improved clinical results, particularly in compromised bone. The potential of such implant surface developments, such as moderately rough surfaces, nanosurfaces, and even bioactive surfaces, also demands separate consideration and will be discussed in chapter 5.

# ROLE OF RELEVANT CELLS IN THE HEALING PROCESS

An *undifferentiated mesenchymal stem cell* is a "cell type which in the adult organism can maintain its own numbers in spite of physiological or artificial removal of cells from the population."[1] In bone, this cell type has a mesenchymal origin and can, after stimulation by growth factors, migrate, proliferate, and differentiate into a more mature form of mesenchymal cell, such as the osteoblast in bone. However, both the nature of the stimuli and the site may cause the stem cells to alternatively differentiate into other types of mesenchymal cells, such as chondrocytes, myoblasts, adipocytes, or fibroblasts.

*Osteoblasts* originate from local mesenchymal stem cells that first develop into preosteoblasts (*osteogenic induction*) and then differentiate into proper osteoblasts. These are densely packed palisade cells on osteoid surfaces and are capable of producing bone; that is, they synthesize, secrete, and regulate the deposition of the extracellular matrix of bone. Osteoblasts produce many different growth factors and have receptors for a wide range of hormones, growth factors, and adhesion molecules involved in cellular attachment. The osteoblasts have cellular processes, later withdrawn in newly formed bone to develop into canaliculi surrounding the daughter cell of the osteoblast, the osteocyte. Osteoblasts, although their function is opposite to that of the osteoclast, work in coupled action with this cell; that is, bone formation and resorption occur at the same sites, such as in so-called creeping substitution of cortical bone.

When osteoblasts have formed bone around themselves, they are called *osteocytes*, the cells of living bone. The osteocytes continue to produce small amounts of matrix proteins on the surface of the noncalcified lacunae that harbor them. The canaliculi, about 1 μm in diameter, connect osteocytes to nearby capillaries, where nutritional elements and cellular influence as well as waste products are transported through diffusion; this mechanism has limited extension, which is why capillaries in bone are found maximally 0.2 mm apart and which explains the formation of the haversian system with ideally organized osteocytes.

*Osteoclasts* are bone-resorbing cells of hematogenic origin, formed by the union of monocytic cells. Osteoclast progenitor cells proliferate and differentiate into osteoclasts after signals from the osteoblastic stromal cells, hormones, and cytokines. The typical location of the osteoclast is on the bone surface, in so-called Howship lacunae, not far from the osteoblasts. The osteoclast is a multinucleated giant cell with several nuclei of various types, heavily influenced by relevant growth factors and hormones.

# ROLE OF GROWTH FACTORS IN THE HEALING PROCESS

Growth factors of bone matrix are called *bone-derived growth factors*. These growth factors are present in the plasma, in very small concentrations of billionths of grams. However, despite the low concentrations, growth factors are important mediators in functions such as cell division, matrix synthesis, and tissue differentiation in every organ system. Different growth factors have their own receptors. Many of the key links in the gene-activating chain of reactions are shared by these groups and therefore sometimes will elicit the same cellular response, despite binding of different growth factors.

The growth factors (proteins, polypeptides) are produced by osteoblasts, nonosteoblastic skeletal cells, and marrow cells and may act systemically or locally to regulate function and growth of cells in several ways. They are located within the bone matrix, which enables dissolution and release after trauma or when prompted by remodeling stimuli. Several growth factors have been found to be stimulated by various types of harmonic influence.

Transforming growth factor β (TGF-β) is a multifunctional peptide with the potential to initiate different biologic activities. It exists in different forms and is produced by osteoblasts and stored in the bone matrix but is also produced by platelets. The bone morphogenetic proteins (BMPs), except for BMP-1, are members of the TGF-β superfamily.

Fibroblast growth factors (FGFs) are believed to have a direct and indirect effect on the recruitment, differentiation, and survival of bone cells during the developmental, postnatal growth, bone-remodeling, and bone repair phases. The FGFs are angiogenic, suggested to induce vascularization during bone healing.

Insulin-like growth factor 1 (IGF-1) and IGF-2, previously often referred to as *somatomedins* (IGF-1) or *skeletal growth factors* (IGF-2), are believed to stimulate not only osteoblastic cells to proliferation and matrix formation but also osteoclast cells to bone resorption. This is perhaps not surprising, because osteoblasts and osteoclasts have a coupled function, despite their opposite mechanisms of action.

Platelet-derived growth factors (PDGFs) are active in fracture healing and implant incorporation. PDGFs are synthesized from cells in the periosteal layer by monocytes, macrophages, endothelial cells, and osteoblasts. Furthermore, there are epidermal growth factors (EGFs), thought by some to be related to TGF-α, that have an influence on angiogenesis, interleukins, and tumor necrosis factors (TNFs) to mention but a few.

Although the importance of various growth factors for proper healing around an implant is evident, this does not necessarily imply that external administration of the same growth factors will produce a more rapid or a stronger bone response. The authors investigated whether administration of growth hormones, FGFs, or BMP-7 could have an effect on implant integration in ordinary stable situations and was unable to verify any contributions to the bone response under such conditions. It also appears that platelet-rich plasma (PRP) placed in combination with particulate bone grafts had no positive effect compared with similar grafts placed without PRP. Nor was it possible to verify any positive effects of PRP with respect to bone regeneration in a peri-implant defect model in dogs.

The drawback of any external administration of growth factors is their rapid turnover; this suggests that some sort of carrier, preferably with a slow-release mechanism, is needed. The proper dosage for external administration has long been discussed, with some remaining controversies. The likely beneficial effect of external administration of growth factors is probably limited to compromised host bone sites, because in a clinical setting, proper controls are rare. Therefore, it is currently difficult to draw reliable clinical conclusions about the true role of externally administered growth factors. At this stage of research development, it is prudent to remain skeptical about the proposed use of oral implants in conjunction with externally administered growth factors, because their efficacy is questionable.

# FUNCTIONAL RECRUITMENT CONDITIONS: TIMING AND LOADING CONCERNS

Implants are placed surgically so that they can be eventually or immediately recruited into functional service via prostheses. The original protocol recommended a two-stage surgery with a 3- to 6-month healing interlude between procedures. The objective sought a minimally disturbed healing process to ensure that the developing osseointegration was not compromised in any manner.

This protocol was gradually regarded as unnecessarily restrictive as clinical reports appeared, describing altered and even immediate loading time frames. These increasing numbers of reports were of varying scientific quality but attest to the feasibility of earlier or even immediate loading scenarios (see chapter 10).

This timing shift in overall treatment duration clearly offers both convenience and fiscal implications and has already led to two major published consensus conference reports. The European conference reported that this approach results in clinical results comparable to those reported for conventionally loaded implants. However, a number of shortcomings in the reviewed reports were conceded, such as research design aspects related to exclusion and inclusion criteria and the fact that only a few studies were controlled and included large enough patient numbers with immediately loaded implants. The North American consensus conference report concluded that the average outcome favored delayed loading, although there were no indications that immediate or early loading cannot be a safe procedure.

## CONCLUSION

Both the literature and clinical experience with short- and long-term healing responses to oral implants suggest the following guidelines:

- The most common reason for short-term disturbed healing is violation of one or more of the six factors listed in Box 2-1 ("Key parameters and determinants of osseointegration"). Clinical experience tends to support the impression that the most commonly encountered violations fall under the headings of departures from, or errors in, well-established surgical and prosthodontic protocols.
- Newcomers to the clinical implant field with limited surgical experience should consider employing a two-stage surgical protocol and a delayed-loading protocol. The surgical novice is likely to produce a more oval and oversized bone defect than the experienced surgeon. This frequently results in implants that are less stable and more prone to movement as opposed to those placed by surgical experts.
- Disturbed healing also may be associated with compromised host sites, such as those with severe bone resorption or previous irradiation. These are very specific surgical challenges and should be managed by qualified surgical experts.
- Modern implant hardware itself rarely causes problems that lead to disturbed healing. However, the apparent current commercial focus on "rapidity and simplicity" may lead to unfavorable responses if new implants are launched without the desired long-term outcome information. It is important that all clinicians insist on scientific credentials for any new implant on the market.

## REFERENCE

1. Lajtha LM. Cellular kinetics of haemopoesis. In: Hardisty R, Weatherall D (eds). Blood and Its Disorders, ed 2. Oxford, England: Blackwell Scientific, 1982: 57–74.

## RECOMMENDED READING

Albrektsson T, Zarb GA, Worthington P, Eriksson RA. The long-term efficacy of currently used dental implants: A review and proposed criteria of success. Int J Oral Maxillofac Implants 1986;1:11–25.

Franke-Stenport V. On Growth Factors and Titanium Implant Integration in Bone [thesis]. Gothenburg, Sweden, University of Gothenburg, 2002.

Frost HM. The biology of fracture healing. An overview for clinicians. 1. Clin Orthop Relat Res 1989;(248):283–293.

Frost HM. The biology of fracture healing. An overview for clinicians. 2. Clin Orthop Relat Res 1989;(248):294–309.

Jokstad A, Carr AB. What is the effect on outcomes of time-top-loading of a fixed or removable prosthesis placed on implant(s)? Int J Oral Maxillofac Implants 2007;22(suppl):19–48.

Nkenke E, Fenner M. Indications for immediate loading of implants and implant success. Clin Oral Implants Res 2006;17(suppl 2):19–34.

Suda T, Takahashi N, Martin TJ. Modulation of osteoclast differentiation: Update. Endocr Rev Monogr 1995;4:266–270.

Thor A. On Platelet-Rich Plasma in Reconstructive Dental Implant Surgery [thesis]. Gothenburg and Uppsala, Sweden: University of Gothenburg and University of Uppsala, 2006.

Triffit J. The stem cell of the osteoblast. In: Bilezikian J, Raisz L, Rodan G (eds). Principles of Biology, ed 1. New York: Academic Press, 1966:39–50.

Trippel S, Coutts R, Einhorn T, Mundy G, Rosenfeld R. Growth factors as therapeutic agents. J Bone Joint Surg 1996;78A:1272–1286.

# Materials, Designs, and Surfaces

Ann Wennerberg | Tomas Albrektsson | Clark Stanford

The material, design, and surface of an implant have long been regarded as important determinants of successful treatment. Implants optimized in these aspects may reduce healing times and thereby improve clinical success. This would certainly impact favorably when immediate or early loading is prescribed.

To date, commercially pure titanium has been the dominant material choice for dental implants. However, other materials with excellent biocompatibility have been employed in implant manufacturing. Some implants are titanium alloy (titanium-aluminum-vanadium [Ti-6Al-4V]), while others have hydroxyapatite (HA) or other calcium phosphate coatings. Good clinical results have been reported in follow-up studies of varying durations.

The major designs used for osseointegrated implants have been cylinders and screws, with the latter design dominant. Numerous variations in screw design with respect to pitch height and thread curvature are available, and it appears that scientific evidence does not favor one design as being significantly clinically better than another (Fig 5-1).

Current implant surfaces tend to be moderately rough and isotropic (Fig 5-2) with the importance of nanometer structures and the effects of chemical modifications becoming of increasing interest. Altering surface topography will most often result in a changed surface chemistry as well, indicating the need to consider different aspects of surface quality rather than topography alone. Available clinical documentation mainly refers to topographic changes at the micrometer level of resolution, although in vitro and in vivo data with a scientific focus on nanosurfaces are now available. In addition, some in vivo and clinical studies have reported on various surface chemical modifications.

The purpose of the various modifications is to stimulate a stronger bone response; in the case of bioactive implants, the goal is to create chemical bonds between the surface and surrounding tissues. Such anchorage would be established rapidly, whereas eliciting an interlocking response through bone ingrowth alone is a time-dependent outcome. According to Hench's 1990 definition, surfaces with potential to create chemical bonds are *bioactive*. However, it is difficult to prove the existence of such bioactivity, because available evidence for its existence is mainly of an indirect nature.

Other authors use the term *bioactivity* to describe a surface with increased ability to stimulate bone-forming cells to produce bone; that is, the surface modification itself results in osseoconduction. If this interpretation of bioactivity is used, in vitro studies using simulated body fluid (SBF) may be a means to assess bioactivity via measurements of the amount of calcium and phosphate precipitation that may occur.

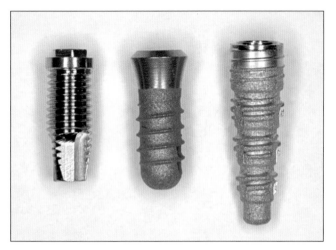

**Fig 5-1** Three screw-shaped commercial implants demonstrating different thread designs *(left to right)*: Lifecore, SLA, Frialit-2.

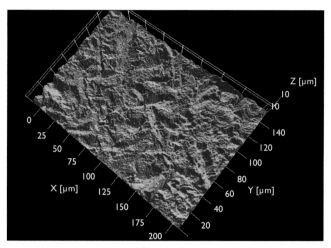

**Fig 5-2** Moderately rough, isotropic implant surface (OsseoSpeed, Astra Tech).

## IMPLANT MATERIAL

The vast majority of oral implants are produced from commercially pure titanium, which is available in four grades. Grade 1 contains the lowest carbon and iron content, while grade 4 contains the highest. The material's mechanical properties significantly improve with increasing amounts of carbon and iron content, with an increase in the titanium's metallurgical physical properties due to changes in grain structure resulting from the addition of low levels of carbon and iron.

Further improvement of the mechanical properties is found for grade 5 titanium—a titanium alloy, Ti-6Al-4V, which is also used for oral implants. For example, yield strengths are approximately 195 N/mm$^2$ for grade 1, 460 N/mm$^2$ for grade 4, and 900 N/mm$^2$ for grade 5, respectively, with corresponding values for tensile strength of approximately 400 N/mm$^2$, 700 N/mm$^2$, and 1,200 N/mm$^2$.

Other materials used include various forms of calcium phosphate coating, commonly referred to as hydroxyapatite (HA). Calcium phosphates are seldom used as solid implants because of the poor mechanical properties of the ceramics and are instead applied as a surface coating. The typical plasma-sprayed HA coatings used in past implant designs had a minimal thickness of 40 to 50 μm. However, the coating often loosened from the underlying bulk metal and caused clinical failures. Today, nanometer-thin coatings with improved adhesion to the bulk metal are becoming more frequent. A coating, regardless of its thickness, will influence the implant's topographic properties.

Clinical studies comparing different materials are really nothing more than very general comparisons of different implant brands. The key point is that implant materials differ together with their likely variations in design and surface topography.

## SURFACE TOPOGRAPHY IN THE MILLIMETER RANGE

Implants used in the oral environment have one of three major types of macroretentive features: screw threads (self-tapping or not), solid body press-fit designs, or sintered bead technologies. Each of these approaches is designed to achieve initial implant stability and/or to create large volumetric spaces for bone ingrowth.

These designs also assist in an important biologic principle of bone—its capacity to respond to compressive loading. Therefore, screw thread designs have been adapted to achieve compressive loading of the surrounding cortical or cancellous bone. For instance, certain implant designs (Straumann) use a 15-degree cutting thread profile to create a compressive interfacial stress. This thread profile has a rounded tip (reducing shear forces at the tip of the tread), which appears to maintain bone in the compressive zone beneath the thread profile.

In an attempt to improve initial bone stability, various implants have been designed to incorporate dual (or more) cutting thread profiles (with or without a screw-based press-fit).

**Fig 5-3** Turned, anisotropic surface.

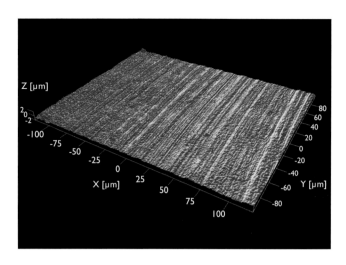

## SURFACE TOPOGRAPHY IN THE MICROMETER RANGE

Two sets of threads cut at different relative locations in the osteotomy as a means of reducing initial stripping (eg, on overseating), which risks loss of primary stability (Mark III, Mark IV, and NobelSpeedy, Nobel Biocare).

Still other thread designs (Microthread, Astra) focus on reducing surrounding cortical bone shear forces by reducing the height of the thread profile (reducing the contribution of any one thread) through an increase in the number of threads per unit area of the implant surface. This design claims the added benefit of increasing the strength of the implant body by increasing the amount of remaining wall thickness of the implant body.

Orthopedic prostheses (eg, femoral stems, pelvic acetabular caps, and knee prostheses) have taken advantage of the macroretentive feature of various sintering technologies to create mesh or sintered beads as a surface for bone to grow into. The application of this technology to dental implants has involved attempts to improve the success rate of short implants (< 10 mm in length), which are conventionally associated with higher failure rates when used with turned surface implant designs. Recent use of short implants (< 8 mm in length) with moderate rough surfaces is also reported as promising. Applying sintered beads to an implant's surface (ie, sintered bead technology) has also led to the development of one commercially available implant system (Endopore, Innova) that shows quite favorable clinical results. A 93% to 100% relative success rate at 3 to 5 years has been reported even for very short implants (7.7 mm) in the posterior maxilla, a site that is popularly regarded as a potentially vulnerable one for implant survival.

Based on current knowledge, implant surface roughness is defined by measuring the average height deviation of the surface irregularities (Sa). *Smooth implants* are those with an Sa value of < 0.5 μm and generally vary between 0.1 and 0.3 μm in roughness, while *minimally rough implants* have an Sa value of 0.5 to 1.0 μm. The latter include turned Brånemark (Nobel Biocare) and Astra Tech implants, acid-etched Osseotite implants (BIOMET/3i), and calcium-reinforced oxidized implants (Ospol). *Moderately rough surfaces* have an Sa value between 1.0 and 2.0 μm; most modern implants are found in this category, which includes TiUnite (Nobel Biocare), TioBlast and OsseoSpeed (Astra Tech), SLA/SLA Active (Straumann), and Cellplus (Dentsply). *Rough implants* are those with an Sa value > 2.0 μm and are exemplified by plasma-sprayed devices such as the Frialit-2 implant (Dentsply).

It is noteworthy that all of the aforementioned surfaces are isotropic; that is, the irregularities are randomly distributed over the entire surface. This is in contrast to the turned anisotropic Brånemark implant surface (Nobel Biocare), which has been regarded as the gold standard for many years (Fig 5-3).

Numerous in vitro studies have demonstrated increased osteoblastic proliferation and cellular differentiation on moderately rough surfaces, and cellular alignment has been demonstrated to be influenced by the surface orientation. However,

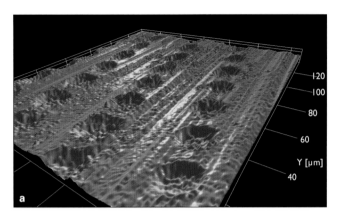 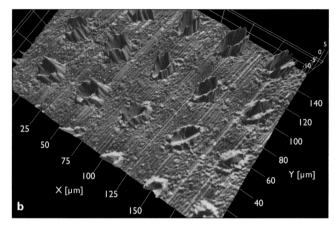

**Fig 5-4** Checked pattern on an implant flank, produced with a photolithography technique *(a)* and a laser technique *(b)*.

direct comparisons cannot be made between results obtained in cell cultures and in vivo observations. In vivo situations are complicated and dependent on interactions between different types of cells, the presence of growth and other hormones, and loading stimuli, to mention but a few important factors. Consequently, it is not possible to compare in vivo experimental results and clinical outcomes due to the even more complicated situation in the latter case.

In a series of rabbit studies performed during the 1990s, it was demonstrated that a blasted implant surface with an average height deviation of about 1.5 µm, an average wavelength of about 11.0 µm, and a surface-developed ratio of 1.5 seemed optimal for firm bone integration. Both minimally rough and rough surfaces showed less strong bone responses than the moderately rough ones over the study's time frame. These observations suggested the possibility of using different clinical time-dependent protocols when different roughened surfaces are selected. Surfaces with randomized irregularities (isotropic surfaces) appear to achieve more enhanced bone fixation than do those with a defined surface orientation (anisotropic surfaces) or surfaces with a checked pattern (Fig 5-4).

It has also been debated whether or not moderately rough surfaces will introduce clinical risks. However, at present, concerns regarding impaired stability and increased ionic leakage do not seem to be incriminating factors for implant failures. An increased incidence of long-term development of mucositis and peri-implantitis has been reported for rough plasma-sprayed surfaces, but has still not been shown for moderately roughened surfaces. However, clinical follow-up studies of more than 10 years are still lacking.

Most reported clinical evaluations comparing minimally rough with moderately rough to rough surfaces suggested no significant difference. However, a general tendency toward better results for the moderately rough implants was noted. Several clinical studies do report significantly better results when patients with poor bone quality and quantity are treated with moderately, rather than minimally, rough implants. In clinical circles, it appears that moderately rough implants present clinical advantages for patients with compromised bone tissue or in challenging situations such as early loading.

## SURFACE TOPOGRAPHY IN THE NANOMETER RANGE

The importance of nanometer surface irregularities continues to be frequently discussed in current biomaterials publications. From a historical aspect, it is noteworthy that so-called micropits, once patented by Brånemark, were regarded as essential for proper osseointegration. Brånemark's micropits were less than 1 µm in size, that is, in the nanometer range.

Several in vitro studies have already shown increased osteoblastic adhesion, osteoblastic proliferation, and differences in protein concentration adsorbed on surfaces with modified nanometer topography.

In addition, in vivo tissue responses to the presence of nanometer-sized indentations with controlled micrometer-sized irregularities are currently being investigated. Electropolished cylindrical test implants in rabbit bone have been compared with nanometer structures coated on the electropolished samples. Some recent laboratory test results indicate that these structures may influence the bone's early healing process.

**Fig 5-5** Particles with an approximate size of 20 nm adhering to an etched implant surface (NanoTite).

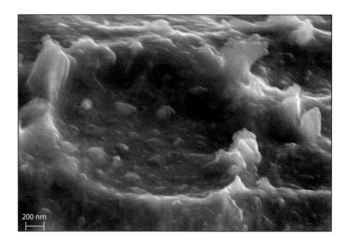

200 nm

Newer surface design for a commercial implant is the Nano-Tite surface (BIOMET/3i). This surface modification is based on nanometer-sized particles of HA coated on the surface, suggestive of a change in the chemistry and the nanometer-level topography (Fig 5-5). Nanostructures have also been identified on the fluoride-etched OsseoSpeed implant (Astra Tech). However, to date, there are no clinical reports that have verified any presumed benefits of nanostructures.

# PHYSICAL AND CHEMICAL SURFACE MODIFICATIONS

Other examples of physical modifications that may influence implant incorporation in the host tissue are surface charge and energy. Hydrophilic surfaces have a high surface energy (and thus a high degree of wettability), in contrast to hydrophobic surfaces. Hydrophilic properties have been regarded as a necessary condition for tissue integration in biomaterials science, yet several modern oral implants, such as the TiUnite and SLA designs, are hydrophobic.

A recently published in vitro investigation reported that high surface wettability was achieved by rinsing samples in deionized water, drying them under nitrogen protection, and finally storing them in an isotonic sodium chloride solution. The increased surface energy, which was speculated to depend on the prevention of contamination in air, demonstrated increased osteoblast alkaline phosphatase and osteocalcin activities that may promote increased bone formation, a conclusion supported by other recent findings in animal studies.

Additional experimental in vivo studies as well as clinical investigations of implants with a high surface energy or hydrophilic properties, however, have been unable to document any advantages of such surfaces. One factor that may have influenced the lack of positive evidence of high surface energy was hypothesized to be an inevitable neutralization of the energy state at implant insertion. To date, the potential contribution to clinical success of particular hydrophilic implants must be regarded as unknown.

Reference is commonly made to *bioactivity*, defined by Hench[1] as "the characteristic of an implant material which allows it to form a bond with living tissues." Examples of biomaterials with assumed bioactivity include calcium phosphate ceramics, titanium treated with alkali and heat, fluoridated titanium implants, and anodized implants in a calcium- or magnesium-containing electrolyte. Implants treated in such manners have demonstrated cohesive fracture in the surrounding bone rather than at the implant interface (adhesive fracture) during attempts at removal; an absence of distinct boundaries between the implant and bone tissue at the ultrastructural level; and otherwise inexplicable differences in bone response from that of controls of identical surface micrometer roughness. However, whether this strong bone response in the individual studies really depends on hydrophilic properties, surface charge, bioactivity, or on other as yet unknown surface physical characteristics remains to be investigated.

Various surface preparations have been evaluated in vitro by using a simulated body fluid model. Immersion of a biomaterial in SBFs, that is, solutions with ion concentrations approximately equal to those of human blood plasma, allows observation of the nucleating capacity of the material. It has been suggested that the nucleation of calcium phosphates mimics

Table 5-1 Summary of properties of commercial implants cited in the text

| Implant* | Mode of surface preparation[†] | Published 1-y clinical results[‡] (> 95% success) | Published 5-y clinical results[‡] (> 95% success) | Published 10-y clinical results[‡] (> 90% success) | Comments |
|---|---|---|---|---|---|
| TioBlast (Astra Tech) | Blasting | Yes | Yes | Yes | |
| OsseoSpeed (Astra Tech) | Blasting + fluoride etching | Yes | No | No | Minor, approximately 1 atomic wt% of fluoride on surface |
| Frialit-2 (Dentsply) | Blasting + etching | Yes | No | No | Stepped, threaded design; rough surface |
| Cellplus (Dentsply) | Blasting + etching + high temperature | No | No | No | |
| Endopore (Innova) | Porous-coated | Yes | Yes | No | Material: Ti-6Al-4V; tapered design; sintered surface |
| Turned (Nobel Biocare) | As-machined with turning process | Yes | Yes | Yes | Minimally rough surface |
| TiUnite (Nobel Biocare) | Anodized | Yes | Yes | No | Phosphate ions on surface |
| Replace (Nobel Biocare) | Anodized | No | No | No | Tapered design |
| Ospol (Ospol) | Anodized | No | No | No | Minimally rough surface; calcium ions on surface |
| SLA (Straumann) | Blasted + etched | Yes | Yes | No | |
| SLActive (Straumann) | Blasted + etched + hydrophilic | No | No | No | |
| Osseotite (BIOMET/3i) | Etched | Yes | Yes | No | Minimally rough surface |
| NanoTite (BIOMET/3i) | Etched + coated with nanoparticles of HA | No | No | No | Material: Ti-6Al-4V; minimally rough surface |

*All implants were threaded screws if not noted otherwise in the "Comments" column. All implants were manufactured of commercially pure titanium, except for Endopore and NanoTite, which were manufactured of Ti-6Al-4V.

[†]All implants were moderately rough, ie, had an Sa value of 1.0 to –2.0 µm, if not noted otherwise in the "Comments" column (minimally rough: Sa 0.5 to –1.0 µm; rough: Sa > 2.0 µm).

[‡]Simple cumulative success rate curves without dropout analyses and bone height measurements do not qualify for success evaluation and were not included.

the initial mineralization of bone on the implant surface. In Kokubo's recently published review, a positive correlation was described between apatite formation in SBF models and in vivo bone bioactivity within the same glass-ceramic material. However, when compared with the SBF model, the in vivo process is more complex, with proteins, enzymes, and biologic factors each playing an important role. So far no clinical documentation is available for bioactive surfaces.

# Biologic Modification of Implant Surfaces

Another technique to create a bioactive surface may be to coat the implant with proteins known to be of importance for cellular adhesion. So far several in vitro studies have shown positive effects, although only few in vivo studies have shown similar results. Since protein adsorption may contribute to cellular behaviors, it has also been speculated that the protein adsorption itself could be responsible for the possible bioactivity of specific materials.

The biomolecules are administered to the implant's surface either by adsorption or by covalent immobilization. Covalent immobilization is hypothesized to provide an opportunity to align and expose the appropriate active site for a more rapid physiologic response. A commonly used technique to covalently attach peptides and proteins to commercially pure titanium surfaces is silanization (amino-functionalization), sometimes with additional coupling agents such as glutaraldehyde.

The covalent coupling of bioactive peptides also includes the possibility of coupling growth factors to the implant surface. Over the past 30 years, a wide assortment of growth factors with a variety of growth-promoting (mitogenic) and bone-inductive (differentiation) activities have been described. However, few studies have dealt with growth factors covalently immobilized to titanium surfaces, and so far there is weak evidence of increased bone response in vitro and in vivo.

It is reasonable to suggest that at this time no clinical documentation is available to support the prescription of biologically modified implant surfaces.

## CONCLUSION

Table 5-1 summarizes properties of commercially used implants mentioned in this chapter, while a literature analysis suggests the following:

- The majority of currently used oral implant systems rely on a combination of commercially pure titanium material, threaded designs, and moderately rough surfaces. There is limited long-term clinical outcome documentation about the use of titanium alloy, HA-coated, and porous-coated dental implants.
- Bioactive and nanosurfaces remain topics of considerable interest, but their effects are to date clinically undocumented.

## REFERENCE

1. Hench LL. Bioactive glasses and glass ceramics: A perspective. In: Yamamuro T, Hench L, Wilson J (eds). Handbook of Bioactive Ceramics, vol 1. Boca Raton, FL: CRC, 1990:7–23.

## RECOMMENDED READING

Albrektsson T, Brånemark P-I, Hansson H-A, Lindström J. Osseointegrated titanium implants. Acta Orthop Scand 1981;52:155–170.

Albrektsson T, Wennerberg A. Oral implant surfaces. 1. A review focusing on topographical and chemical properties of different surfaces and in vivo responses to them. Int J Prosthodont 2004;17:536–543.

Baier RE, Meyer AE, Natiella JR, Natiella RR, Carter JM. Surface properties determine bioadhesive outcomes: Methods and results. J Biomed Mater Res 1984;18:337–355.

Kokubo T, Takadama H. How useful is SBF in predicting in vivo bone bioactivity? Biomaterials 2006;27:2907–2915.

Meirelles L. On Nanostructures and Enhanced Bone Formation [thesis]. Gothenburg, Sweden: Gothenburg University, 2007.

Mustafa K, Wennerberg A, Wroblewski J, Hultenby K, Silva Lopez B, Arvidson K. Attachment, proliferation and differentiation of cells derived from human mandibular bone to titanium surfaces blasted with $TiO_2$ particles. Clin Oral Implants Res 2001;12:515–525.

Nanci A, Wuest JD, Peru L, Brunet P, Sharma V, Zalzal S. Chemical modification of titanium surfaces for covalent attachment of biological molecules. J Biomed Mater Res 1998;40:324–335.

Pilliar RM. Overview of surface variability of metallic endosseous dental implants: Textured and porous surface-structured designs. Implant Dent 1998;7:305–314.

# DIAGNOSTIC IMAGING

MICHAEL J. PHAROAH | ERNEST W. N. LAM

Diagnostic imaging is inarguably an essential adjunct in assessing the selection of host bone sites for implant placement. However, imaging that employs ionizing radiation carries a risk and a cost. Therefore, the prescription of imaging must be based on the clinical examination, a determination of the type of information required, and an evaluation of the radiation risk-benefit ratio for the patient. Consequently, use of the most advanced imaging modality may not always be appropriate. For instance, the application of computerized tomography (CT) for the analysis of potential implant sites in a severely atrophic maxilla with negligible bone available for implants is exposing a patient to unnecessary radiation and cost, when a less sophisticated imaging modality may have provided the necessary information.

An imaging examination can contribute significant information to the preoperative assessment of the jaws prior to implant placement. It can determine the vertical and horizontal dimensions of existing bone of the maxilla and mandible, the outer contours of the jaws, the density of trabeculation of the cancellous component, the thickness of the outer cortical plate, the positions of internal vital structures such as the inferior alveolar canal, and the health of the bone. While intraoral radiography still provides the greatest image detail for viewing bone architecture and the health of the adjacent dentition, cross-sectional imaging is the most accurate method of obtaining the dimensions, outer contour, and positions of internal vital structures for the analysis of specific potential implant sites.

The advent of cone-beam computerized tomography (CBCT) has greatly facilitated this analysis; moreover, this technique imparts a significantly lower dose of radiation to the patient than does medical CT. Actual bone density can be measured

using quantitative CT or dual-photon absorptiometry; however, bone density has not been shown to have a significant influence on the success or failure of dental implants.

This chapter provides an analysis of the application, strengths, and weaknesses of various imaging modalities for implant treatment planning.

## PANORAMIC RADIOGRAPHY

The panoramic image is a useful starting point for initial assessment of potential implant sites because it displays all of the osseous structure of the maxilla and mandible in one image. Furthermore, the determination for the need and the type of advanced imaging should be based on the initial findings of this radiograph. For instance, if the panoramic image reveals approximately 2 to 3 mm of vertical bone in the maxilla, there is no need to proceed with sophisticated cross-sectional imaging (Fig 6-1).

Panoramic radiography provides information on the approximate locations and dimensions of structures such as the maxillary antra, nasal fossae, and inferior alveolar nerve canals. It also provides a rough estimate of the amount of atrophy of the alveolar processes of the maxilla and mandible. The panoramic image can also provide evidence of pathologic conditions of the jaws, the status of the dental structures, and a rough depiction of the internal density of the bone of the jaws, but this is limited by overlapping images of adjacent structures. Panoramic imaging is also readily available, and it delivers relatively low patient radiation doses.

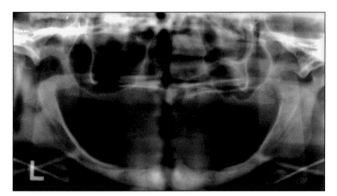

**Fig 6-1** Panoramic image revealing the lack of adequate vertical bone height for the placement of maxillary implants.

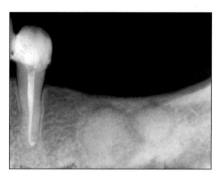

**Fig 6-2** Periapical radiograph revealing the presence of two regions of cemental dysplasia.

The major weaknesses of panoramic imaging include substantial image distortion, the generation of phantom or ghost images, and the inability to depict the buccal and lingual contours of bone. Image distortion is variable throughout the panoramic image, and has been measured to be up to 25%, with errors as great as 3 mm, thereby limiting the usefulness of such measurements.

Although measurements made in the vertical dimension are less susceptible to distortion than measurements made in the horizontal dimension, no such measurements are meaningful unless there is a standard of known dimension positioned exactly in the region of interest. For instance, placing a metallic marker on the crest of the alveolar process exactly at the point of the intended measurement during the imaging procedure can provide an object of known dimensions within the panoramic image. If the magnification of the image of the marker is determined and then applied to a measurement made in the vertical dimension through the marker, the result may be more meaningful.

For the same reason, it is also not possible to reliably determine the locations of vital anatomic structures such as the position of the inferior alveolar canal or distances such as the floor of the maxillary antrum to the crest of the alveolar process.

Overlapping structures, such as the image of the cervical spine, can obscure anatomic detail in the anterior maxilla and mandible. In some cases, this overlap may even suggest the presence of a pathologic condition.

Finally, the panoramic image provides no detail about the buccal or lingual surface contours such as the submandibular gland fossa, the sublingual gland fossa, and the incisive fossa of the mandible or the canine fossa and incisive fossa of the maxilla.

# Intraoral Radiography

The intraoral radiograph delivers very low radiation dose, has a low cost, and is readily available. Because these films still produce images with the greatest spatial resolution and detail, intraoral radiography is useful when detail regarding the internal structure of the bone or adjacent dental structures is required. For instance, the differentiation between a dense bone island and cemento-osseous dysplasia is important and requires an image with good spatial resolution (Fig 6-2). Moreover, the diagnosis of pathoses related to tooth structures may require the detection of very subtle changes in the lamina dura or periodontal membrane space. In the postoperative setting, periapical radiography may be particularly useful in assessing peri-implant healing or the identification of peri-implant pathoses.

Depending on the vertical angulation of the incoming x-ray beam, there may be variability in the accuracy of vertical measurements. The use of standardized film holders, however, may lessen variability of image geometry from one examination to the next (Fig 6-3). The major disadvantage of the intraoral periapical projection is that it cannot provide information in the third dimension, that is, in the buccolingual dimension.

Occlusal radiographs have been employed for investigations of the mandible to obtain more information in the buccolingual dimension. These images should be used with caution, because the buccal and lingual contours of the mandible are not uniform as a result of the presence of convex curves and concavities of the outer bone surfaces (Fig 6-4). Therefore, the occlusal radiograph may provide a false perception of maximum width of the mandible, superimposing wider buccolingual regions over narrower ones. The curvilinear contours of the mandible are particularly evident in the regions of the sublingual and submandibular gland fossae.

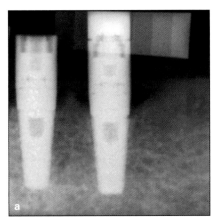
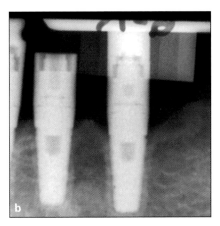

**Fig 6-3** *(a and b)* Two periapical images made 1 year apart with a film-holding device. Note the consistent image geometry of the attached implant.

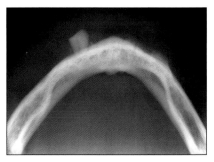

**Fig 6-4** Occlusal projection revealing two lingual cortical plates in the premolar regions due to a substantial sublingual gland fossa.

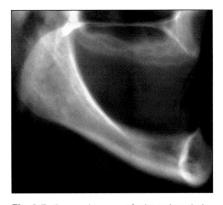

**Fig 6-5** Cropped image of a lateral cephalometric radiograph. The apparent cross-sectional image actually represents only the midline region of the mandible and maxilla.

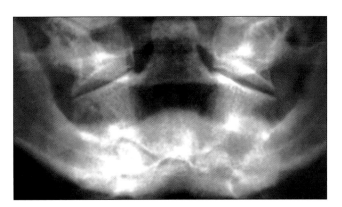

**Fig 6-6** Cropped image of a posteroanterior cephalometric film, revealing the vertical height of the anterior segments of the maxilla and mandible.

# CEPHALOMETRIC RADIOGRAPHY

Like panoramic and intraoral radiography, cephalometric radiography delivers a comparatively low dose of radiation and is readily available. In a standard lateral cephalometric setup, a predictable head position is obtained using a craniostat, and the distance from the source of radiation to the plane of the image receptor is precisely controlled; hence image magnification is minimized and can be accurately predicted. This is the basis of cephalometric measurements used in orthodontic treatment.

Lateral skull and posteroanterior skull cephalometric images have also been employed in preoperative implant imaging.

Although the lateral cephalometric view provides an opportunity for some cross-sectional analysis, this is restricted to the most anterior aspect of the mandible and maxilla (Fig 6-5). This portion of the image is actually an average of the midline and perimidline regions only and does not provide information in the canine region. This information can be supplemented by the image of the posteroanterior skull view, which will provide a lingual to buccal view of the anterior maxilla and mandible, providing information regarding variations in the vertical height (Fig 6-6).

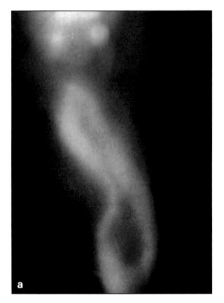
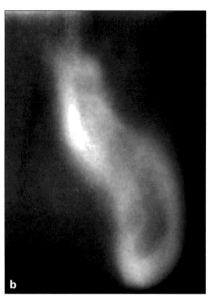
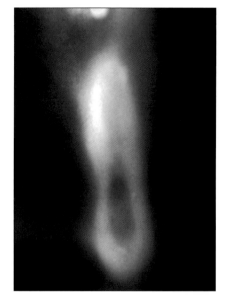

**Fig 6-7** *(a and b)* Two tomographic image slices revealing substantial sublingual and submandibular fossae that dramatically reduce the width of the mandible.

**Fig 6-8** Tomographic image revealing the inferior alveolar canal and the fact that the mandible has a thin buccolingual dimension.

# CONVENTIONAL TOMOGRAPHY

In the past, conventional tomography was the most commonly used form of cross-sectional imaging for preoperative implant analysis. This technique is based on the principle that objects located outside of a tissue plane defined by a moving source of radiation (x-ray tube) and the image receptor during the exposure appear blurred. The motion of the x-ray source and image receptor may be in one direction (referred to as *linear tomography*), or in multiple directions (referred to as *polydirectional* or *complex motion tomography*). The most common type of polydirectional tomography uses a hypocycloidal motion.

The thickness of the plane of tissue imaged can be controlled by the complexity of motion. Moreover, the orientation of the image plane relative to the maxilla or mandible can be controlled by varying the position of the patient's head within the imaging device. In modern tomographic machines, the position of the imaging device and hence the orientation of the image slice to the jaws is computer controlled.

Conventional tomography can provide accurate vertical and horizontal measurements, if the images are of good quality. It has been reported, however, that up to 20% of tomographic studies are not of adequate quality. The orientation of the image slice will determine the accuracy of vertical and horizontal measurements. Therefore, the slice must be oriented at right angles to the horizontal axis of the portion of the jaw that is being imaged as well as the buccal and lingual cortices of bone.

Measurements made using conventional tomography are more accurate than those made using intraoral or panoramic images; however, the accuracy of measurements is strongly influenced by the quality of the images and inherent image blurring. In research using dry skulls, the measured error of conventional tomography is less than 1 mm. In a cadaver study using spiral tomography, the vertical measurement error to the inferior alveolar canal ranged from 0.10 to 1.05 mm.

Tomographic image slices depict the outer contours of the jaws and can show variations because of the positions and locations of the submandibular, sublingual, canine, and incisive fossae (Fig 6-7). Also, the positions of internal structures such as the maxillary sinuses, nasal fossae floors, and inferior alveolar canals can also be revealed. A clear view of the canal depends on the direction of the x-ray beam relative to the long axis of the canal (Fig 6-8) and the density of the surrounding trabecular bone. The cortices of the canal are best seen when the tomographic slice is acquired at right angles to the course of the canal. In some patients, however, there may not be enough contrast between the canal and the surrounding bone to accurately locate the canal.

**Fig 6-9** Cross-sectional reconstructions through the maxilla generated from reconstructed medical CT images. The panoramic image at the top indicates the positions of each cross section in the maxilla.

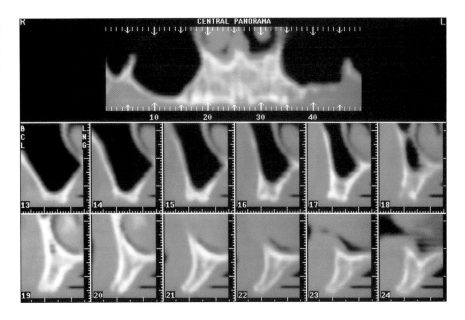

Locating the anterior wall of the maxillary sinus is also problematic, because this cortical boundary is not at right angles to the x-ray beam. Teeth with large metallic restorations produce profound radiopaque artifacts within the image that may hide detail in adjacent image slices.

Conventional tomography may also be used to monitor bone graft material, sinus-lift procedures, and repositioning of the inferior alveolar canal.

In comparison with panoramic and intraoral radiography, conventional tomography delivers higher doses of radiation to the patient. However, compared with medical CT, doses from conventional tomography are generally less, except for complete-arch examinations. Unfortunately, conventional tomography is not readily available and has a greater cost than panoramic or cephalometric examinations. In many centers, conventional tomography is being replaced by CBCT.

# MEDICAL AND CONE-BEAM COMPUTERIZED TOMOGRAPHY

Medical CT was first used as an alternative to conventional tomography when bone measurements from multiple implant sites were required. The main advantage of this modality over conventional tomography was the ability to obtain cross-sectional images at multiple sites in a substantially shorter period of time. In addition, the greater contrast of these images enabled better visualization of bone graft material.

In medical CT, patients are placed in the supine position on a motorized CT gantry bed. The patient is then fed through an aperture around which a fan-shaped x-ray beam moves. A series of detectors that line the open aperture captures the radiation exiting the patient, and complex algorithms are used to reconstruct the image from the detected radiation.

To create cross-sectional images of the jaws using medical CT, thin-slice axial images are first acquired. This acquisition may take several minutes to complete, and the patient must remain stationary during this time. These axial images are then "stacked" and the data are reformatted so that buccolingual cross sections are created perpendicular to a line that matches the curve of the maxillary or mandibular dental arch (Fig 6-9).

To optimize resolution of the reformatted images, it is important to minimize both patient movement and slice thickness of the original axial images. Patient movement as well as thicker axial image slices produce step patterns along the reconstructed bone borders that may be unacceptable.

To ensure measurement accuracy of the reformatted cross-sections, it is important to acquire the original axial images

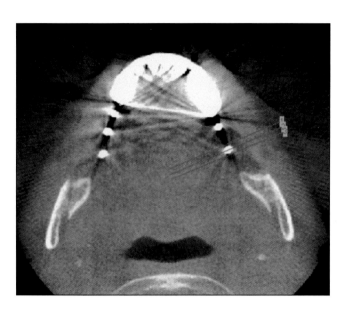

**Fig 6-10** Axial CBCT image showing five radiopaque markers and the positions of three reconstructions (labeled 1 to 3) through the mandible.

along an axis oriented at right angles to the horizontal axis of the portion of the jaw that is being imaged. For imaging purposes, most hospital radiology departments will position their patients on the CT gantry bed so that the Frankfort horizontal plane is aligned parallel to the plane of the CT unit and perpendicular to the plane of the floor. This orientation may not produce images along the correct axis but may generate oblique cross-sectional images.

One final, but significant, drawback of medical CT is the substantial radiation absorbed by the patient.

In a CBCT examination, the patient may be seated upright or be supine, depending on the type of system being used, and the patient remains stationary. A cone-shaped x-ray beam rotates around the patient during image acquisition, which is complete in less than 1 minute. The orientation of the patient is not vital, because reconstruction software can be used to reorient the patient's jaws in a position that will minimize distortion of the reconstructed images (Fig 6-10). The most substantial advantages of CBCT over medical CT are access and availability, acquisition time, and radiation doses that are fractions of medical CT radiation doses.

Several reconstruction paradigms are available for medical or cone-beam CT data, the choices of which may be system specific. Most systems will, however, enable the user to define the size of the field of view of the reconstruction as well as the slice thickness and interslice intervals (the distance between the centers of individual images) around the arch (Figs 6-11 and 6-12). Narrower slices (0.5 or 1.0 mm) may be chosen over thicker ones (2.0 or 3.0 mm), and the same choices can be made for interslice intervals.

Thicker slices may be more susceptible to volume-averaging artifacts that may mask the variation of crestal bone height across an implant site, while thin slices may not adequately reflect variations of crestal bone height unless multiple regions of the edentulous space are sampled. Although the rationales for choosing a particular slice thickness or interslice interval are arbitrary, these variables should be discussed by and agreed on by the radiologist and surgeon at the time of imaging.

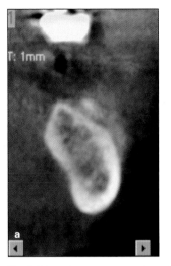 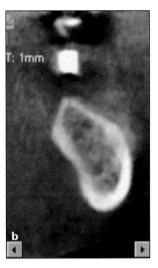 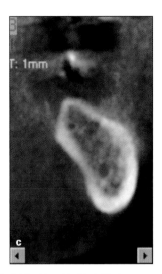 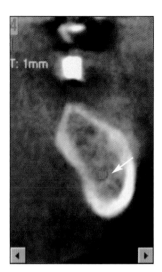

**Fig 6-11** CBCT cross sections through the left posterior region of the mandible. *(a)* Position 1 in Fig 6-10, the most mesial cross section. *(b)* Position 2 in Fig 6-10. *(c)* Position 3 in Fig 6-10, the most distal cross section.

**Fig 6-12** CBCT cross section in the same location as Fig 6-11b, showing the position of the mandibular canal *(arrow)*.

## Imaging Stents

The accurate measurement of bone dimensions and the transfer of these measurements to the surgical site can only be done if radiopaque markers are incorporated in the tomographic image. This usually entails the fabrication of an occlusal splint in which markers are incorporated in the regions of the potential implant sites. Furthermore, it may be useful to incorporate markers that indicate the angulation at which the implant will be introduced to the bone. That way, any guesswork related to the orientation of the bone measurements can be minimized or altogether eliminated.

## Imaging Software

All cone-beam imaging systems have proprietary software that enables the user to create cross sections of the jaws and perform measurements. Additionally, there are several third-party sources that accept Digital Imaging and Communications in

Medicine (DICOM) data from CBCT systems to facilitate surgical planning and surgical splints using three-dimensional models.

## Conclusion

The rationale for prescribing an imaging procedure prior to dental implant placement rests on the necessity to locate the positions of vital anatomic structures within the jaws prior to implant placement and to capture subtle curvatures of the buccal and lingual surfaces of the maxilla or mandible. The locations and positions of the air spaces of the maxilla and the mandibular neurovascular canal system may limit implant lengths, while variations in the contours of the mandible and maxilla may restrict implant orientations and limit implant diameters. Each imaging technique has advantages and limitations; the optimal imaging technique must be selected individually for each patient, based on the clinical examination, the type of information required, and the radiation risk-benefit ratio.

# RECOMMENDED READING

Bou Serhal C, van Steenberghe D, Quirynen M, Jacobs R. Localisation of the mandibular canal using conventional spiral tomography: A cadaver study. Clin Oral Implants Res 2001;12:230–236.

Eckerdal O, Kvint S. Presurgical planning for osseointegrated implants in the maxilla. Int J Oral Maxillofac Surg 1986;15:722–726.

Grondahl K, Ekestubbe A, Grondahl H-G. Radiography in Oral Endosseous Prosthetics. Gothenburg, Sweden: Nobel Biocare, 1996:27–32.

Lam EWN, Ruprecht A, Yang J. Comparison of two-dimensional orthoradially reformatted computed tomography and panoramic radiography for dental implant treatment planning. J Prosthet Dent 1995;74:42–46.

Ludlow JB, Davies-Ludlow LE, Brooks SL, Howerton WB. Dosimetry of 3 CBCT devices for oral and maxillofacial radiology: CB Mercuray, NewTom 3G and i-CAT. Dentomaxillofac Radiol 2006;35:219–226 [erratum 2006;35:392].

Reddy MS, Mayfield-Donahoo T, Vanderven FJ, Jeffcoat MK. A comparison of the diagnostic advantages of panoramic radiography and computed tomography scanning for placement of root form dental implants. Clin Oral Implants Res 1994;5:229–238.

Schulze D, Heiland M, Thurmann H, Adam G. Radiation exposure during midfacial imaging using 4- and 16-slice computed tomography, cone beam computed tomography systems and conventional radiography. Dentomaxillofac Radiol 2004;33:83–86.

Sonick M, Abrams J, Faiella RA. A comparison of the accuracy of periapical, panoramic, and computerized tomographic radiographs in locating the mandibular canal. Int J Oral Maxillofac Implants 1994;9:455–460.

Stella JP, Tharanon W. A precise radiographic method to determine the location of the inferior alveolar canal in the posterior edentulous mandible: Implications for dental implants. 1. Technique. Int J Oral Maxillofac Implants 1990;5:15–22.

Stella JP, Tharanon W. A precise radiographic method to determine the location of the inferior alveolar canal in the posterior edentulous mandible: Implications for dental implants. 2. Clinical application. Int J Oral Maxillofac Implants 1990;5:23–29.

Tal H, Moses O. A comparison of panoramic radiography with computed tomography in the planning of implant surgery. Dentomaxillofac Radiol 1991;20:40–42.

Truhlar RS, Morris HF, Ochi S. A review of panoramic radiography and its potential use in implant dentistry. Implant Dent 1993;2:122–130.

# 7

# SURGICAL CONSIDERATIONS

GERALD BAKER | DAVID J. PSUTKA | LESLEY DAVID

The initial application of the Brånemark osseointegration phenomenon was directed to support fixed-detachable restorations for completely edentulous patients who could not otherwise manage removable denture prostheses. Planning for these cases was based on clinical and routine radiographic examinations.

At that time, when teeth were extracted, implant placement was deferred for several months until there was evidence of postextraction bone regeneration. Buccal incisions were used to facilitate wide exposure of the alveolar ridge and ensure primary coverage for the underlying implant and cover screw. Sequential drilling protocols were initially employed with multiuse, but subsequently single-use, burs of increasing dimensions. Bone tapping and countersinking were routinely required prior to the complete submergence of the implant and cover screw.

The early implants were straight-walled, single-threaded, and non–self-tapping screws of nonalloyed commercially pure titanium that had a machined, visibly smooth surface. They were left submerged for 4 to 6 months and then exposed through crestal incisions for the attachment of permanent straight healing abutments. Attachment of a plastic healing cap allowed placement of a periodontal dressing to compress the mucosa, assisting in the mucosal attachment phenomenon. Typically, 6 weeks of mucosal healing was the norm before initiating the prosthetic restorative phase.

Forty years later, implant-supported prostheses are the tooth replacement technique of choice in most cases. Techniques have evolved, and there has been a great increase in numbers and types of implants and instruments available. Implant protocols include those for the single tooth, multiple missing teeth, complete edentulism, maxillofacial reconstruction (including eye or ear prosthetic attachment to specialsized implants), and hearing restoration. There have been a variety of incision modifications, including flapless surgery in selected cases. Accelerated treatment schedules have evolved, including implant placement at the time of extraction in specific situations and single-stage surgery in good quality bone where primary stability is achieved, thereby obviating the need for a second operation. Predictable hard and soft tissue reconstruction techniques have evolved to optimize implant site anatomy. Protocols exist for immediate transitional prostheses and, in some cases, early definitive prostheses.

Design changes to the implant itself may support a simplified surgical procedure and enhance primary stability by supporting an earlier osseointegration process. These include selftapping screw designs, tapered designs, multiple thread patterns, and various surface treatments such as rough surfaces, microgrooving, and crestal minithreads. Newer complementary technology, such as narrow one-piece implant systems, zygomatic implants, ultrashort implants, and provisional implants, in specific situations and in expert surgical hands, may expand the available strategies for managing anatomically challenging situations.

Virtually every edentulous anatomic region may become an implant site because of the myriad surgical and prosthetic solutions available. The provider who uses evidence-based procedures combined with experience and sound judgment and who reconciles a planned intervention, including careful treatment planning, with its outcome potential will thereby offer excellent patient care with a predictable treatment outcome.

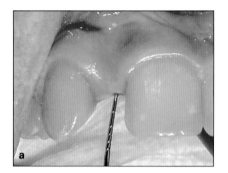 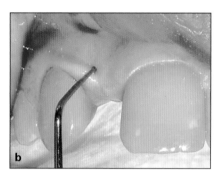

**Fig 7-1** *(a and b)* Sounding the depth of the mucosa to determine bone levels. This can also be done on the palate.

## TREATMENT PLANNING

### History and clinical examination

Treatment planning begins with the patient's medical history, which should include a history of the proposed implant site in order to obtain information that will provide insight as to the potential underlying bony anatomy. For example, long-term edentulism at the site, a congenitally missing tooth, or history of trauma, periodontal disease, or other pathologic condition in that region often implies compromised or even inadequate bone volume. The surgeon would then rely less on a clinical impression of adequate ridge width, perhaps masked by soft tissue thickness, and more on the radiographic assessment. A history or evidence of parafunctional activity will influence surgical planning, such as the numbers of implants to be used, and also have prosthetic implications.

The clinical examination is performed and includes an assessment of the patient's smile line, soft tissue health and characteristics, pathologic conditions at the intended implant site or areas immediately adjacent, ridge relationships, general dental health, excessive occlusal attrition, occlusion, muscle attachments, buccal depth, and mouth opening. Specific to the site in question, the clinician must consider the status of adjacent teeth; visible or palpable crestal irregularities; buccal, labial, or lingual concavities; the adequacy of interdental and interarch space; and soft tissue quality, thickness, and contour.

Underlying bony architecture may be assessed by bone-sounding procedures (Fig 7-1). This requires probing the buccal and lingual regions of the edentulous space in conjunction with measuring the ridge thickness, allowing the surgeon to determine soft tissue thickness, osseous ridge width, and the presence of bony concavities.

### Cast analysis

In conjunction with clinical examination, cast analysis helps determine ultimate prosthetic and surgical requirements, including specific anatomic challenges often less evident during clinical assessment. Mounted casts with a diagnostic waxup may emphasize important ridge deficiencies as well as assist in the identification of the most ideal site for implant placement driven by specific prosthetic requirements, irrespective of adequate bone volume. When osseous deficiencies become evident, the surgeon may consider reconstructive procedures.

The diagnostic waxup may be used to fabricate an implant placement guide to help optimize implant placement (Fig 7-2). Visualization of the cervical margin and labial-buccal and lingual outlines of the proposed restoration as indicated in a surgical and prosthetic template allows appropriate positioning of the implant in all three dimensions of space. This in turn results in both an esthetic and appropriately loaded restoration. Ideally, the implant should be submerged 2 to 3 mm apical to the cervical margin of the proposed implant restoration if normal gingival marginal levels are present. Implant depth will be adjusted if there is adjacent gingival recession and if it is warranted due to the soft tissue biotype (see chapter 8).

An implant placement guide may also be used when bone augmentation is performed prior to implant placement. This allows for anatomically correct and adequate bone augmentation.

Cast analysis, diagnostic waxups, and surgical templates also permit assessment of adequate space requirements for prosthetic components. For example, in the completely edentulous patient with adequate bone height, deeper placement of the implants, implying a surgical alveolectomy or alveoplasty, may be required to create space for the prosthetic hard-

**Fig 7-2** Three different implant placement guides: groove cut into the buccal surface *(a)*; palatal acrylic resin removed and the buccal facing preserved *(b)*; central cingulum channel cut into the acrylic resin *(c)*. *(d)* Direction indicator sitting within the implant placement guide to ensure proper implant placement.

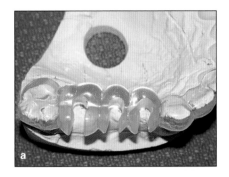
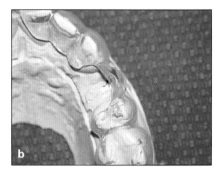
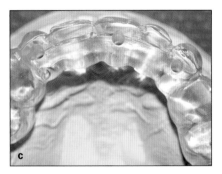
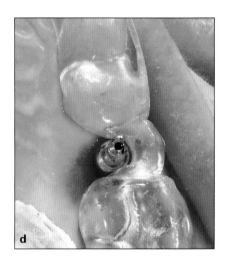

ware and/or to mask the transition between a hybrid type of prosthesis and the underlying ridge in a patient with a high smile line. In the esthetic zone, with single-tooth replacement, however, caution must be exercised in such a surgical maneuver because the resultant bone loss and soft tissue adaptation from deeper implant placement may result in compromised esthetics.

## Diagnostic imaging

Radiographic examination is the ultimate presurgical means of determining underlying bone quantity and perhaps quality (see chapter 6). Significant anatomic structures in the surgical field can also be visualized. This information will more readily allow the surgeon to differentiate the more routine from the complex surgical cases. The synthesis of clinical and radiographic findings with the preferred prosthetic plan guides the surgical protocol.

In single or partially edentulous situations, high-quality, undistorted, periapical radiographs are useful because they confirm interradicular space and identify bone height, pathologic conditions, and adjacent anatomic structures. Bone levels on teeth adjacent to the edentulous area must also be vi-

sualized. In the esthetic zone, this bone level determines the ultimate presence or absence of the interdental papilla. It also determines the amount of predictable vertical bone augmentation that can be achieved in the event that a vertical bone defect is present. Other imaging may be required if it is not possible to obtain accurate periapical views.

A panoramic radiograph is useful in both the completely and partially edentulous patient because it demonstrates the arches in their entirety as well as pertinent anatomic structures. High-quality panoramic views will assist in measurement of bone height more accurately in the posterior zones than in the anterior zones, particularly in the maxilla. In taking measurements, the surgeon must recall that panoramic radiographs are magnified (typically by 25%) compared with a properly taken periapical view.

A lateral cephalometric radiograph may be useful to supplement a panoramic radiograph because it allows visualization of maxillary and mandibular midline (but not lateral to the midline) morphology (Fig 7-3). Moreover, this view will emphasize the relative maxillary and mandibular positions in the sagittal plane, an important consideration in determining whether surgical repositioning or reconstruction procedures are needed if poor anatomic relationships will compromise the intended prosthetic result.

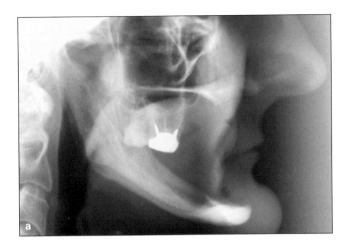

**Fig 7-3** Extreme maxillary and mandibular atrophy revealed by lateral cephalometric *(a)* and panoramic *(b)* radiographs.

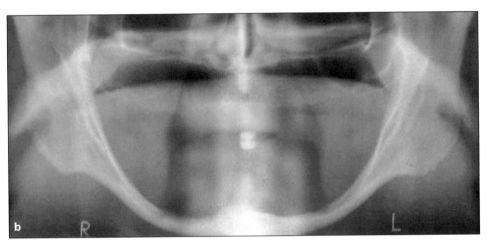

Regardless of the plain radiograph taken, the surgeon must adequately visualize the maxillary sinus, floor of the nose, mental foramen, and inferior alveolar nerve if implants are to be placed at or near these anatomic sites. If plain radiographs are inadequate, adjunctive imaging is needed. Conventional tomography and cone-beam computerized tomographic (CT) scans are very helpful (Fig 7-4). These very detailed studies allow the radiologist to reconstruct cross-sectional anatomy demonstrating ridge contours as well as both the quantity and quality of bone. Surgical templates with radiographic markers can also be used during the imaging process to relate existing bone anatomy to the ideal restorative and implant placement sites.

Three-dimensional reconstructed images may also be generated using different software programs that enable virtual implant planning, including precise, computed-generated implant placement guides that allow extreme precision during implant surgery. This technique will be discussed later in this chapter.

CT imaging may also provide insight into bone density. An appreciation of relative amounts of trabecular and cortical bone will assist in determining if any modifications are necessary for the planned surgical procedures.

Radiographic analysis enables visualization of a particularly important area when considering anterior mandibular implant surgery: the mandibular lingual concavity (see Fig 6-4). Cadaver studies of the anterior mandible have shown three different bony morphologies that may be encountered: *(1)* the mandible progressively widens from the crest to the inferior border both labially and lingually; *(2)* the labial and lingual plates are parallel and may tilt lingually; or *(3)* a concavity is noted lingually in the middle to inferior region of the mandible. Implant surgery may not be possible in mandibles with the second configuration without surgical reconstruction. Cavalier site preparation in patients with the second or third type of configuration could lead to perforation of the lingual cortex, resulting in significant intraoperative and postoperative bleeding from damage to adjacent perforating vessels arising from both the lingual and submental arteries. Lack of recognition and failure to manage this promptly will result in hematoma formation and potential life-threatening airway compromise.

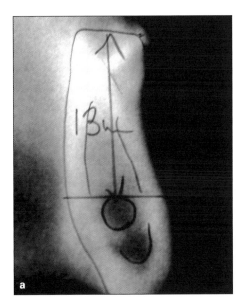
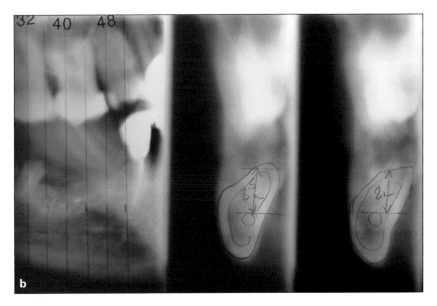

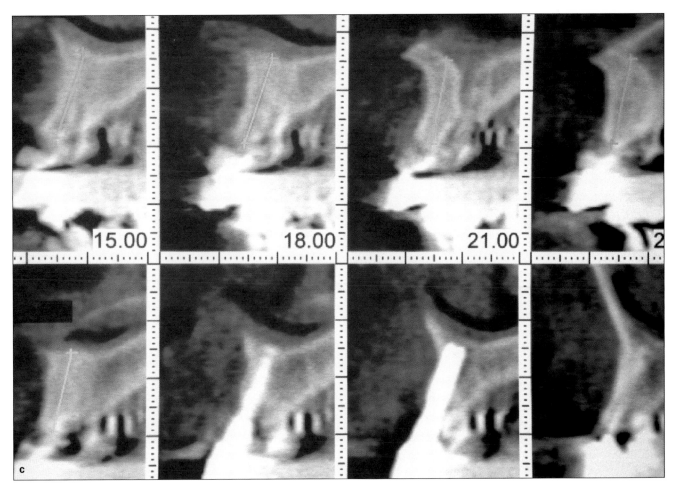

**Fig 7-4** *(a and b)* Cross-sectional CT allowing accurate measurement from the alveolar crest to the mandibular canal. These images demonstrate bone height from the "ideal" crestal position of the planned implant to the top of the mandibular foramen. *(c)* Cross-sectional SimPlant (Materialise Dental) cone-beam CT images of the maxillary anterior anatomy, from which accurate measurements can be taken.

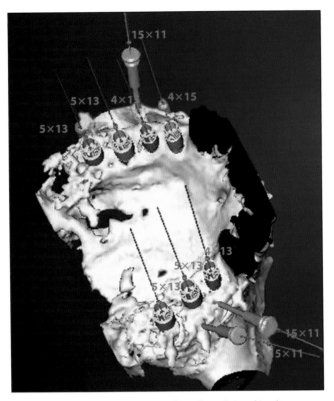

**Fig 7-5** Three-dimensional image of maxilla and virtual implants.

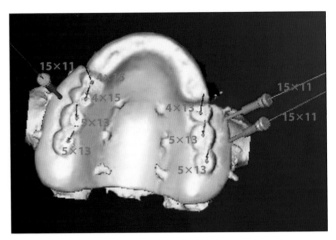

**Fig 7-6** Prosthesis visualized on a three-dimensional image, enabling restoratively driven implant placement.

## SURGICAL PROTOCOL

Knowledge of the prosthetic treatment plan enables restoratively driven implant placement. This, in turn, determines any hard and soft tissue surgical reconstruction or modification procedures required for ideal implant placement in support of the intended results.

The basic surgical protocol for implant placement requires the use of a series of sequentially enlarging twist drills, used with copious saline irrigation in a slow and purposeful entry into and exit out of bone, to create an intrabony osteotomy into which an implant is placed. The implant preparation is slightly smaller than the diameter of the implant, whose threads then cut into the bone walls, providing initial stability. In some implant designs, the implant is "press fitted" into the bone preparation.

The quantity and quality of bone and the anatomy of the overlying soft tissue determine the extent to which surgical variation from this basic protocol may be needed. Because pri-

mary implant stability is required for predictable osseointegration, the basic bone preparation may have to be modified if bone quality is inadequate. For example, type 4 bone (very loose textured marrow with little cortical bone) offers poor mechanical stability (see Fig 1-16). Surgical maneuvers designed to improve initial stability may include underpreparing the osteotomy site, preparing the site using a variety of osteotomes rather than twist drills to compact the bone, and/or gaining primary anchorage in adjacent cortical bone. In some cases, the surgeon may also elect to eliminate the countersinking step required of some implant designs.

The procedure may also have to be modified in very dense, mainly cortical, type 1 bone typical in the anterior mandible, particularly in the severely resorbed edentulous patient. The decreased vascularity of such bone leaves it more susceptible to overheating during the twist drill preparation, and more caution is required to assure the availability of viable bone required for the osseointegration process. The surgeon must use

**Fig 7-7** *(near right)* Custom surgical template (implant placement guide) with three fixation sites and with embedded metal cylinders to allow for precise implant placement.

**Fig 7-8** *(far right)* Surgical template rigidly fixed to the maxilla with implants in place.

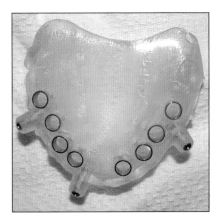
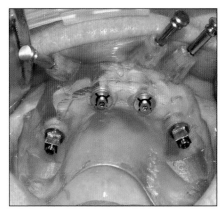

**Fig 7-9** Panoramic view of ideally situated implants using computer-generated planning procedures.

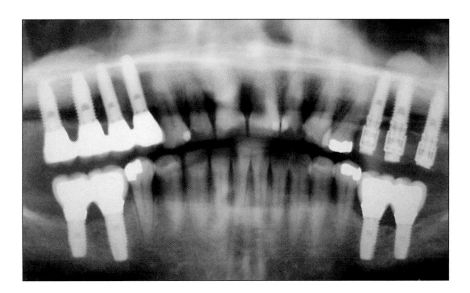

new and therefore very sharp twist drills, with more irrigation to maintain a temperature of less than 47°C, for less than 1 minute. It usually is prudent to prethread (tap) the site. The surgeon must never use excessive force, which may exceed recommended torque values during implant insertion.

## Surgical templates

Newer CT software programs enable virtual implant planning so that the clinician places virtual implants in a three-dimensional reconstructed model of the edentulous site (Figs 7-5 to 7-9). The prosthesis is also visualized so that implants can be placed according to the proposed restoration. One software program then enables fabrication of a custom surgical template that is used for the surgery and can be used to preoperatively fabricate the patient's prosthesis. A provisional or definitive prosthesis may be generated by using the surgical template to pour a final cast with implant analogs on which the prosthe-

sis can be made. The restoration is delivered immediately, once the implants have been placed, if immediate loading is both desired and appropriate. Insertion torques recommended for immediate loading are 35 to 45 N/cm.

The custom surgical template is rigidly fixed to the arch at the beginning of the implant placement procedure. Flapless surgery ensues in most cases. The surgical template has sleeves incorporated in it; drill guides, fitting intimately into the surgical template sleeves, are used for the osteotomy preparation. The use of such drill guides enables precise implant placement according to the presurgical planning. This, in turn, may allow for immediate prosthetic rehabilitation with the prefabricated prosthesis. It would seem prudent, in most circumstances, to place provisional rather than definitive restorations if immediate rehabilitation is undertaken.

The surgical template may also just be used to facilitate the surgical procedure without prosthesis fabrication and immediate loading. The advantages cited with the use of such a template are easy and precise implant positioning, less invasive surgery (because a flapless technique is usually employed), and a significant reduction in surgical time. Empirically, this usually results in decreased postoperative swelling and pain and a more rapid postsurgical recovery.

A potential disadvantage is the use of the flapless protocol in instances where there is a lack of keratinized tissue in the proposed implant sites. There is no suggestion in the literature, however, that there is greater long-term implant survival if implants are surrounded by keratinized tissue. Nonetheless, soft tissue quantity and quality are of paramount importance in the anterior esthetic zone, and, as such, a flapless technique in this area should be used cautiously and only when there is an adequate band of keratinized gingiva. In cases where preservation of keratinization is desired, the protocol may be modified, and a conventional flap technique may be employed while using these surgical templates. Given the intimate fit of the instrumentation and the flapless technique, irrigation of the surgical field can be restricted. Heat generation secondary to inadequate cooling results in bone necrosis and lack of osseointegration. When preparing the osteotomy site using these surgical templates, the surgeon must be diligent to ensure adequate entry and exit with the twist drills, enabling delivery of adequate irrigation to the twist drills and, in turn, the bone.

The key to success with computer-guided implant treatment is proper planning and adherence to meticulous surgical procedures predicated upon basic biologic principles. A thorough understanding and application of both the prosthetic and surgical steps must be adhered to for successful outcomes. This may not be a procedure for the novice implant surgeon.

# RESIDUAL RIDGE RECONSTRUCTION

Dental implants must be placed into bone of adequate quantity and quality (density) to ensure predictable osseointegration. This biologically based process requires vascularized, osteocyte-rich bone. Bone loss in the maxilla and mandible may be secondary to disuse atrophy, metabolic disorders, trauma, periodontal inflammation, maxillary sinus expansion, long-term denture wear, and pathologic conditions. The rates and patterns of bone resorption following tooth loss in the maxilla and mandible have been well described. Essentially, resorption occurs in both the vertical and horizontal dimensions.

Where presurgical planning has demonstrated bone of inadequate volume, it is possible to reconstruct the anatomy using various surgical procedures with bone or bone substi-

tutes. Careful planning and adherence to basic biologic and surgical principles will help assure successful reconstruction. Reconstruction procedures are technique sensitive and can be complicated by infection, graft dehiscence, and resorption.

## *Materials*

### Grafts

The decision as to which bone graft material to use among the many available can be quite challenging for the implant surgeon (Box 7-1). Understanding the inflammatory, proliferative, and resorptive remodeling phases of bone healing assists the surgeon in making a decision (see chapter 4). This information also helps explain the observation that grafted bone that does not subsequently receive implants in a timely fashion will ultimately resorb, unless the graft is of a nonresorbable material.

***Autogenous bone grafts*** Autogenous bone is nonimmunogenic and transfers freshly obtained viable osteogenic cells, facilitating osteogenesis. It also has associated osteoinductive and osteoconductive capabilities (both phase I and phase II bone graft healing), making it the gold standard of bone grafting materials (Box 7-2 and Table 7-1).

Autogenous bone is harvested in the form of corticocancellous blocks or particulate grafts. The block grafts can be contoured to create various sizes and shapes as needed. They are then stabilized to the donor site with screws. Particulate bone grafts are condensed, packed into defects, and contained by bony walls or surgical membranes. Condensing particulate grafts is thought to increase the population of transplanted bone-forming cells, thus increasing the potential for more dense bone formation. Small volumes of autogenous bone can be harvested from intraoral sites such as the ramus, chin, tuberosity, or zygoma (Fig 7-10). Harvesting of intraoral bone adds minimally to the morbidity of the grafting procedure, especially in cases where the graft is harvested adjacent to the recipient site. The dense cortical bone of the mandible is typically type 1 or 2. It resorbs slowly and minimally, providing for predictable ridge augmentation. The symphysis and ramus grafts can provide corticocancellous blocks of varying thickness, typically 4 to 6 mm. The maxillary tuberosity, the zygoma, and implant osteotomy sites also provide particulate bone, which can be collected in a suction trap.

Intraoral bone harvesting is convenient but nevertheless warrants advanced training and experience. The ramus bone-harvesting procedure can be complicated by injury to the inferior alveolar nerve and fracture of the coronoid process and/or mandibular angle. Symphyseal bone harvests have been complicated by injuries to teeth, damage to the incisive

**Box 7-1** Materials for alveolar ridge reconstruction

- *Autogenous bone:* Bone harvested from the patient
  - Extraoral: Iliac crest, rib, fibula, tibia, calvarium
  - Intraoral: Mandibular ramus, chin, maxillary tuberosity, zygoma
- *Allograft:* Donor bone
  - Freeze-dried, demineralized, or mineralized bone
- *Xenograft:* Anorganic bone
  - Animal source (bovine, porcine)
- *Alloplast:* Artificial bone substitutes
  - Resorbable or nonresorbable

**Box 7-2** Types of bone formation

- *Osteogenesis:* Primary bone formation through the direct transfer of living bone cells
- *Osteoconduction:* Growth of bone along a surface through the placement of a graft that acts as a scaffold for creation and maintenance of a new space and an appropriate conduit for inbound migration of blood vessels and bone-forming cells from the wound periphery
- *Osteoinduction:* Transfer of bioactive mediators (osteoinducers, osteopromoters, or bioactive peptides) that stimulate the differentiation of stem cells to become bone-formers

TABLE 7-1 Phases of bone healing

| Phase | Name | Activity |
|---|---|---|
| Phase I | Steady-state phase | Preosteoclast transformation to osteoclasts |
| Phase II | Resorption phase | Resorption of graft, 8 d |
| Phase III | Inversion phase | Macrophagic debridement |
| Phase IV | Formation phase | Osteoblast bone synthesis, 80 d |
| Phase V | Quiescence phase | Bone remodeling, maturation |
| Bone graft vascularization | — | 30 d |
| Bone graft remodeling | — | 90 d |

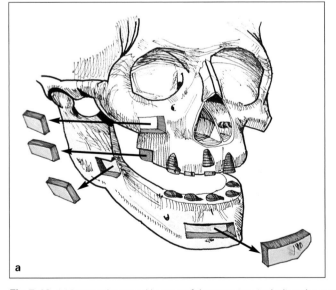

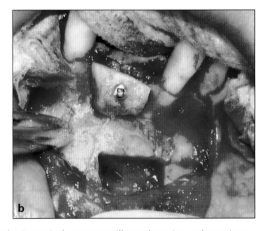

**Fig 7-10** *(a)* Potential intraoral bone graft harvest sites, including the symphysis, vertical ramus, maxillary tuberosity, and anterior zygoma. *(b)* Bone harvested from the symphysis and grafted to an alveolar ridge that has a labiolingual deficiency. The graft is rigidly fixed with a bone screw and will remain so during 6 months of bone graft healing.

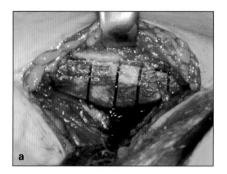

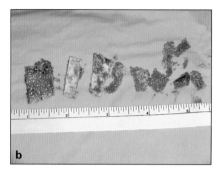

**Fig 7-11** *(a)* Bone harvested from the inner table of the anterior iliac crest. *(b)* Strips of corticocancellous bone from iliac harvest. *(c)* Graft rigidly secured to residual maxillary alveolar bone. *(d)* Implants placed 6 months later.

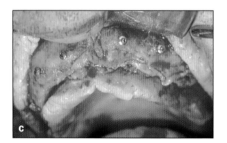

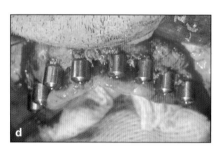

branch of the inferior alveolar nerve, and bleeding from the lingual artery with resultant severe hematoma formation and airway compromise. Tuberosity harvests may result in inadvertent oroantral communication.

Extraoral sites allow harvesting of larger volumes of bone. The rib, calvarium, ilium, and tibia are all potential donor sites. The iliac crest is the most common donor site for larger amounts of bone (Fig 7-11); on average, 20 to 25 cm³ of bone can be harvested from the anterior crest, and 50 cm³ or more can be harvested from the posterior crest. Corticocancellous blocks and particulate grafts are readily harvested from these sites. This is an advanced procedure performed by experienced oral and maxillofacial surgeons. Iliac crest bone harvest can be performed routinely on an outpatient basis, although large volume harvests or associated medical comorbidities may warrant an overnight stay in the hospital. Mild to moderate hip pain and gait disturbance are common but transient postoperative sequelae. Infection, anterior iliac spine fracture, bleeding, and thigh numbness are rare complications.

***Allografts*** The desire to avoid a second surgical site to acquire autogenous bone has lead to the widespread use of bone graft substitutes, either alone or in conjunction with autogenous bone. Bone allografts, alloplasts, and xenografts, which may act as graft expanders when used in conjunction with autogenous bone, are osteoconductive, providing a slowly resorbing scaffold for the inbound migration of host pluripotential osteogenic cells from the wound periphery (phase II bone graft healing) or from the added autogenous graft cells.

Allografts and xenografts are the most commonly used graft alternatives, although both have slightly increased risks of immunogenic reaction and infection and neither heal as predictably as autogenous bone. These materials take longer to resorb and, therefore, require longer healing times (4 to 6 months for autogenous bone versus 6 to 9 months for allogeneic or xenogeneic bone). The fear of disease transmission (for example, bovine spongiform encephalopathy, human immunodeficiency virus, and prion-related disease such as Creutzfeld-Jakob disease) has underscored the importance of sterilization in graft preparation. To date there has not been a single reported case of serious disease transmission using these materials, which speaks to the efficacy of current tissue-processing techniques.

Human donor bone (allograft) is procured in a sterile manner from screened cadavers and processed to remove potentially immunogenic organic matrix, leaving only the mineral components. Mineralized grafting material is solvent dehydrated and finally gamma irradiated for sterility.

Allografts may have varying degrees of osteoinductive capability. The demineralization of allograft bone by host osteoclasts or by the preparatory process (as in freeze-dried demineralized bone grafting material) exposes organic noncellular bone matrix, releasing various biomolecular inducers, such as bone morphogenetic protein (BMP), that transform host progenitor cells into osteoblasts. Several variables can negatively influence the osteoinductive capacity of the BMP, including donor age and factors in tissue processing (retrieval method, time, and temperature, and sterilization technique such as gamma irradiation).

**Fig 7-12** *(a)* Xenograft (Bio-Oss) and alloplast (DynaGraft, Isotis) mixed with autogenous bone harvested from a bone suction trap and placed over exposed threads at the implant sites. *(b)* Particulate bone harvested from a bone suction trap. *(c)* Teflon insert (DuPont) that traps the bone material.

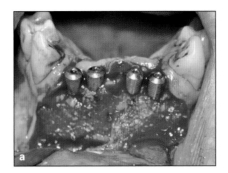
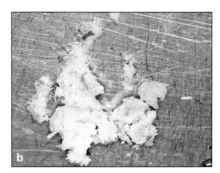
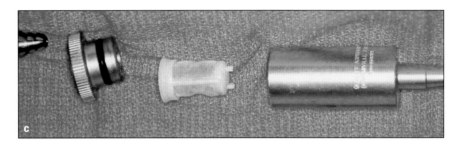

Consequently, clinical results with processed demineralized bone have been mixed. Allograft bone is available in mineralized or demineralized formats. Many surgeons prefer mineralized allografts, which resorb more slowly, maintaining the volume of the expansion more predictably.

Allografts are most commonly available as particulate grafts, which lend themselves to being mixed with autogenous bone and packed into walled defects, the maxillary subsinus region, or fresh extraction sockets. However, allograft corticocancellous blocks have recently become commercially available, although they are quite expensive. Such grafts may obviate the need for autogenous block graft harvest procedures. Their efficacy has been reported favorably in a few limited case report studies. Further clinical study is warranted to understand their long-term efficacy.

**Xenografts** The widespread availability and low cost of xenografts (tissue derived from other species) makes their use for implant site development appealing. They are prepared as deproteinized particulate inorganic mineral scaffolds. Bio-Oss (Osteohealth) is a commonly used bovine-derived material favored for its human bone–like porosity. The bone is chemically treated to remove its organic components. It is then heated to 300ºC, maintaining the exact trabecular architecture and crystalline content, while the size of the mineral particles is doubled. Graft porosity encourages angioneogenesis (vascular ingrowth), necessary for the transport of osteogenic cells into the graft.

Xenogeneic materials are also slow to resorb. This can be advantageous in helping to maintain graft volume and strength while phase II bone graft healing occurs (osteoclast resorption of graft material with generation of host osteocytes and osteoid). This slow resorption necessitates longer healing times. A common surgical observation is that xenograft material, rather than living host bone, is still visibly abundant at the time of implant placement even 12 months after grafting. The total time for osseous replacement of Biocoral (Biocoral), derived from the exoskeletons of marine coral, is about 18 months.

Varying results with xenograft materials have prompted some to recommend that this material be mixed with autogenous bone, especially for larger defects (Fig 7-12).

**Alloplasts** Alloplastic bone substitutes may appeal to some surgeons and patients because, like allografts, alloplasts do not require a separate donor site, and there is no potential for disease transmission. Alloplasts must be biocompatible and easy to sterilize, have a microporosity similar to that of bone, and must ultimately resorb. Alloplasts are solely osteoconductive and must be mixed with autogenous bone to impart any osteoinductive capability.

A variety of materials, both synthetic and naturally derived, have been used; these include various forms of ceramic, hydroxyapatite, bioactive glass, calcium sulfate, and tricalcium phosphate. Biostite (Colletica) is a synthetic hydroxyapatite granule in a collagen and chondroitin sulfate carrier. HTR polymer (Lorenz) is a microporous synthetic bone grafting material that combines a polymethyl methacrylate core with a polyhydroxyethyl methacrylate surface, resulting in a biocompatible resin composite. There are many case reports suggesting success with all of these materials, although incomplete resorption, variable replacement by bone, and poor mechanical strength are reported shortcomings. Incomplete resorption may impair implant stability. In general, successful cases have been reported when significant existing bone was available to primarily anchor the implants and when healing times were at least 9 to 12 months. Long-term prospective studies with large sample sizes are lacking.

***Selection criteria*** Current selection criteria for graft materials include the size and location of the defect. Small-to-medium defects (2 to 5 mm) with three or more bony walls heal predictably with allografts or xenografts (possibly mixed with autogenous bone). Defects requiring onlay grafts or larger osseous defects are more predictably reconstructed with autogenous grafts.

Numerous studies have been undertaken in an effort to identify the ideal grafting material, taking into account the ease of access to the graft material, the healing response, and patient morbidity. Lack of agreement regarding the best material was noted in the findings of the 1996 Sinus Graft Consensus Conference, which examined outcome data from multiple centers for bone grafting to the floor of the sinus. Overall, the consensus conference found high success rates with most materials, the exception being freeze-dried demineralized bone used as a sole graft material or to augment other materials.

## Osteoactive agents

An osteoactive agent is any material that has the ability to stimulate the deposition of bone. These biomolecules have been described as *osteoinducers*, *osteopromoters*, or *bioactive peptides*. These include growth factors, morphogens, and mitogens. The reader is referred to chapter 4 for an in-depth review of osteoactive agents.

***Bone morphogenetic protein*** BMP is a naturally occurring protein molecule with osteoinductive properties. Human, bovine, porcine, and various recombinant human (rhBMP) forms of BMP have been developed. Numerous case reports and university-based research theses have demonstrated startling bone generation using BMP or rhBMP alone or delivered to the recipient site on various carriers, including biodegradable gels, collagen sponge, silica glass, hydroxyapatite, and allogeneic bone. A form of rhBMP is commercially available and, in Canada, is approved for use in spinal fusion surgery. It is very expensive, currently costing more than Can\$4,000 for enough material for one subsinus graft procedure. This is not yet a mainstream surgical option, although efficacy in bone formation has been reported. The potential for more cost-effective production of recombinant DNA technology makes this a very interesting future therapy.

***Other bioactive agents*** Transforming growth factor $\beta$ (TGF-$\beta$), platelet-derived growth factor (PDGF), and other bioactive polypeptides attract ongoing interest because of their ability to stimulate or enhance bone formation. Collection of these biologic materials, their high-volume manufacture at a reasonable cost, and provision of substrate vehicles on which these materials are delivered to the surgical site continue to be practical challenges to clinical application.

***Stem cells*** Tissue engineering for bone generation continues to explore the possibility of seeding biomaterial carriers with osteocompetent cells. Human bone marrow contains stem cells that have the potential to differentiate into various cell types, including bone-forming cells. Coral scaffolds seeded with cells from autogenous bone marrow have been used experimentally to generate mature bone. Such "hybrid grafts" may reduce the need for and morbidity of graft harvesting in the future.

***Platelet-rich plasma (PRP)*** PRP is an autogenously derived concentration of human platelets in a small volume of plasma. The patient's blood is harvested at the time of surgery. Using specially designed centrifuge units, blood is spun down and platelet-rich plasma, platelet-poor plasma, and red blood cells are separated and collected in tubes. Centrifuge technology has evolved so that some commercially available machines facilitate in-office production of PRP. Spinning concentrates the platelets, ideally, to 4 or 5 times normal.

Clotting is initiated by adding bovine thrombin (US protocol) or autogenous platelet-poor plasma (Canadian protocol). The PRP is immediately applied to surgical wounds, including bone and soft tissue grafts. The clotting process creates a gel that congeals the graft material for additional support. This process concentrates the seven protein growth factors actively secreted by platelets, thereby stimulating osteoprogenitor cells and angiogenesis, initiating and driving graft and wound healing:

1. PDGF-$\alpha\alpha$
2. PDGF-$\beta\beta$
3. PDGF-$\alpha\beta$
4. TGF-$\beta$1
5. TGF-$\beta$2
6. Vascular endothelial growth factor (VEGF)
7. Epithelial growth factor (EGF)

PRP also contains fibrin, fibronectin, and vitronectin, cellular adhesion proteins that enhance osteoconduction and act as a matrix for bone, connective tissue, and epithelial migra-

**Fig 7-13** *(a and b)* Rigidly fixed autogenous cortical onlay grafts to increase the width of deficient alveolar ridges. In both cases, bone was harvested from the vertical ramus.

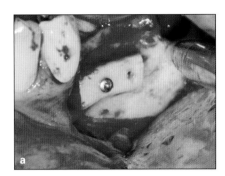
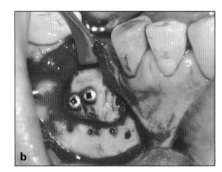

tion. The clotting process activates platelet degranulation and bioactivation of these growth factors. Platelets continue to secrete these growth factors during their normal 7-day life cycle.

Clinical experience and numerous case reports and reviews support the claim that the use of PRP accelerates soft tissue healing. Although it is only a subjective observation, incisional and soft tissue flap healing 1 week postoperatively typically has the appearance of healing that would have occurred after 3 to 4 weeks. Proponents of PRP use in bone grafting believe that bone healing is also accelerated, providing more rapid healing and enhanced bone graft quality (bone density and maturity). Some have suggested this should result in accelerated timing for implant placement into grafted bone and enhance the potential for successful outcomes. Dissertations by some authors strongly support the use of PRP in bone grafting and implant surgery. However, there have also been numerous anecdotal and published experimental and clinical reports concluding that PRP has little or no benefit in healing of bone grafts and long-term outcomes of implant surgery. Some centers that initially used PRP in bone graft surgery have currently abandoned the technique because of a lack of obvious long-term benefit. It has been suggested that these variable outcomes may be the result of poor PRP collection technique, the use of ineffective centrifuge machines, and the use of homologous or stored blood rather than fresh autogenous blood. Others have observed significant long-term resorption in grafts that have been treated with PRP. It has been proposed that this phenomenon could result from concentrating the antiangiogeneic and resorptive biomediators that are also present in platelet granules. The use of PRP continues to be considered a controversial adjunctive strategy in many centers and is not presently a universally practiced modality. Further clinical study should bring greater clarity to the indications and expected clinical outcomes for PRP.

## Surgical techniques

### Onlay bone grafts

Lateral augmentation of the residual alveolar ridge with onlay bone grafts is generally quite predictable, while vertical augmentation is more challenging, regardless of the technique employed. The maximum extent of vertical augmentation is limited to the bone level on the roots of adjacent teeth in partially edentulous individuals. Appropriately shaped blocks of autogenous bone are adapted to prepared recipient sites to facilitate intimate interfacial contact. Rigid fixation with 1.5-mm titanium screws prevents graft micromotion, which would result in graft resorption or loss. Bone grafts have to be thick enough to cover the planned implants by at least 1.5 mm. Augmentations of 6.0 to 7.0 mm are feasible with this technique.

Some cases lend themselves to simultaneous implant and graft placement, although the implants need to be at least partially anchored in host bone for the required initial implant mechanical stability. The most predictable results in managing large defects are achieved with staged surgery; implants are placed 4 to 6 months following an autogenous bone graft procedure. If allogeneic bone or alloplasts are used, graft-healing times should be extended (Fig 7-13).

Brånemark, in the 1960s, originally suggested the possibility of simultaneous autogenous cortical-cancellous onlay grafts and implant surgery, but these procedures were mainly abandoned because of overall unpredictable long-term success. There are now reports suggesting accelerated time frames may be effective after only 2 months of graft healing; however, the follow-up is short; studies with at least a 5-year follow-up are still required. In general, such accelerated procedures are not recommended, except when patient-specific circumstances warrant it and the patient is in the hands of experienced surgeons.

Tension-free closure of mucosal flaps and provisional restorations that do not directly contact the grafted sites are critical to success. Smoking and systemic medical conditions with known impact on wound healing, such as uncontrolled diabetes or previous radiation therapy to the maxillofacial region, can negatively affect graft healing. Infrequent but potential complications include graft infection, wound dehiscence, resorption, partial or complete graft loss, excessive bleeding, and sensory nerve injury. Fracture of the fixation screw head during the required screw removal can be bothersome if the fractured screw is at the site of the intended implant position. In general, various reports suggest success rates (where the outcome is a healed graft with a subsequently osseointegrated implant) between 80% and 99%.

A variation of onlay grafting for the completely edentulous mandible involves placing a rib graft or an allogeneic mandibular crib with autogenous particulate bone on the inferior aspect of the mandible through a bilateral submandibular or midline submental incision. Implants are placed secondarily a minimum of 4 months later; resorption rates have been reported at less than 5% over several years.

## Membrane-guided bone regeneration

Originally conceptualized and applied to long-bone healing in the late 1950s, the guided bone regeneration (GBR) technique was applied to periodontal regeneration in the early 1980s and alveolar ridge reconstruction for dental implant surgery in the late 1980s. Biologic principles necessary for predictable bone regeneration include:

1. Primary, tension-free soft tissue closure to ensure undisturbed wound healing and prevention of barrier contamination
2. Angiogenesis to provide necessary blood supply and undifferentiated mesenchymal cells
3. Space maintenance or creation to facilitate adequate space for bone ingrowth
4. Avoidance of direct pressure on the wound (and implant) to protect the underlying blood clot and promote uneventful healing

Guided bone regeneration involves the use of biologic or alloplastic barriers to create protected compartments in the area of bone defects that require volumetric augmentation. The barriers prevent ingrowth of unwanted fibroblasts and epithelial cells while promoting the ingrowth of osteoprogenitor cells from the bony walls of the protected defect. The barriers are stabilized with small tacks, screws, or sutures. The desired volume of augmentation can be maintained with autogenous, allogeneic, xenogeneic, or resorbable alloplastic bone grafts or by support screws, which act like tent poles.

Barrier materials may be nonresorbable and bioinert, such as Gore-Tex (expanded polytetrafluoroethylene, WL Gore), Silastic (Dow Corning), or titanium mesh. Titanium-reinforced Gore-Tex membranes are popular because they can be shaped to the desired ridge contour and will not flatten or deform. These barriers are usually left in place for 6 months and are removed at implant surgery. Potential complications include wound dehiscence and subsequent infection, which necessitate premature removal. If this occurs within the first month of healing, the result will usually be compromised. If these barriers are placed simultaneously with implants, they require a second surgery for their removal.

Resorbable membranes are made of synthetic materials such as polylactic acid or polyglactin mesh. Biologically derived materials have included allogeneic dura mater and periosteum or xenogeneic collagen. Xenogeneic collagen membranes are commercially available and variously prepared chemically to increase cross-linking of collagen molecules. Non–cross-linked collagen resorbs within weeks and does not work predictably in GBR protocols, while some of the cross-linked collagen products take up to 6 months to resorb. These materials are favored by some surgeons because they do not require a second procedure for removal and dehiscence rarely necessitates membrane removal.

GBR procedures are technique sensitive but may, in experienced hands, facilitate augmentations of up to 10 mm. Variations of the GBR procedure are used for ridge reconstruction, osseous defect management, antral floor grafting, and tooth socket grafting. Numerous long-term studies have been performed and subsequently reviewed. When appropriate surgical techniques are used, implants placed in alveolar ridges where local defects have been corrected with GBR techniques have survival rates similar to those of implants placed in native bone (Fig 7-14).

## Alveolar osteotomies

Cases of severe alveolar loss in the transverse dimension can be managed with ridge-splitting procedures if the vertical dimension is adequate and there is at least 3 mm of bony thickness. The procedure may be staged so that implants are placed later, or, if primary stability is possible, the implants may be placed immediately.

Mucosal incisions are made well lateral to the ridge crest, in the vestibule or even the buccal mucosa. Blood supply to the labial bone segment is maintained with a supraperiosteal dissection to the alveolar crest, where the periosteum is then incised. Subperiosteal dissection then exposes the crest. Drills and osteotomes split the ridge transversely; vertical and (in the case of dense bone) basal horizontal labial cortical osteotomies serve as stop cuts. The outer cortical bone segment is then "bent" labially to the desired width.

**Fig 7-14** Use of particulate xenograft and resorbable guided tissue regeneration membrane over the exposed threads of an implant placed immediately following extraction of the central incisor.

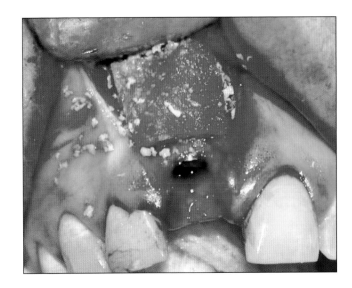

Implants may then be placed if there is adequate apical bone for stabilization. Bone grafts of choice are placed in the gap, and the flap is advanced crestally; mucosa is sutured to the exposed periosteum. Potential complications include fracture or vascular compromise and subsequent loss of the labial bone segment.

## Interpositional bone grafts

Interpositional grafting can be used for vertical augmentation. This technique lends itself to larger segments (at least three or four teeth) where width is good, but vertical height is less than 7 mm. Buccal mucoperiosteal incisions provide access for labial or buccal and lingual or palatal cortical osteotomies, creating a free segment. The crestal and lingual or palatal mucosa is not elevated, because this supplies vascularity to the osteotomy segment. It is this vascularity that minimizes the potential for resorption and loss of the graft. Segment elevation is crestal and stabilized with a cortical block graft, which is placed in the osteotomy defect. Particulate grafts are packed around the site, and implants are placed 4 to 6 months later.

The elastic quality of the lingual or palatal flap tends to rotate the osteotomy segment lingually or palatally. A beveled crestal cut and the use of mini–bone plates can be helpful in managing this problem, if the vector of rotation is inappropriate for the planned implant placement.

A special version of interpositional grafting is the total maxillary osteotomy (Le Fort I maxillary osteotomy) with interpositional bone graft. This may be considered in cases of severe resorption and allows vertical augmentation of the maxilla both anteriorly and posteriorly. In addition, the maxilla may be repositioned in the horizontal plane, and transverse ridge discrepancies may be addressed when required.

With the pattern and nature of bone loss inherent to severe resorption of the maxilla and mandible, there tends to be a resultant Class III maxillomandibular skeletal relationship. Rehabilitation in patients with significant skeletal discrepancies can result in large lateral prosthetic cantilevers. Interestingly, this does not typically result in negative outcomes, as seen in patients rehabilitated with zygoma implants and appropriate occlusal schemes. One may, however, choose to correct these skeletal discrepancies via the Le Fort I osteotomy in which the maxilla is anteriorly repositioned in conjunction with interpositional bone augmentation.

This procedure was introduced in the late 1980s and involves a downfracture of the edentulous maxilla and placement of multiple corticocancellous block grafts in the nasal floor and maxillary sinus or placement of a single horseshoe graft. Autogenous iliac crest (posterior or anterior) is most commonly used. Implant placement may be done at the time of the Le Fort osteotomy or preferably delayed until bony healing has occurred. More predictable and successful outcomes have been reported with delayed implant placement.

Disadvantages of this technique include variability in bone graft healing, relapse potential, and potential donor site morbidity after the autogenous graft is harvested.

## Maxillary sinus floor grafting

Atrophy and pneumatization of the maxillary sinus commonly create bone volume deficits in the posterior maxilla that impede routine dental implant placement. Extensive use of the sinus-lift procedure since the late 1970s and reports of high success rates and low morbidity have made this procedure a widely accepted adjunct to maxillary implant therapy.

Maxillary sinus anatomy is variable. This sinus can extend from the lateral incisor region to the posterior maxilla. The lateral nasal wall is lined by the three turbinate bones, with the osteomeatal complex, or drainage portal of the sinus, residing in the middle meatus. The patency of this opening is crucial to normal ventilation and drainage of the sinus. Graft placement must avoid obstruction of the osteomeatal complex.

The sinus is lined by ciliated pseudostratified columnar epithelium; the cilia suspend mucus secreted from goblet cells in the membrane. The cilia clear the sinus by propelling the mucus toward the osteomeatal complex. This membrane can be exceedingly thin, making surgical manipulation challenging. The preoperative workup should rule out preexisting sinus pathosis such as infection or mucus retention cysts, which can further complicate surgery.

The classic technique for antral floor grafting involves mucoperiosteal flap exposure of the lateral posterior maxilla. A window osteotomy is created in the lateral bony wall, the sinus membrane is judiciously elevated, and the grafting material is placed (Fig 7-15). Numerous modifications in technique, timing, treatment sequencing, and graft materials have been proposed (Table 7-2).

Sinus floor grafting procedures may be complex. The sinus frequently contains small bony septa that divide the sinus into smaller compartments, making membrane dissection difficult. On such occasions, and at other times, the membrane, needed to help confine the graft material, can tear.

Small tears appear to have little or no impact on graft healing. Redundancy of the sinus membrane may allow it to fold on itself, creating a seal. Medium-sized tears may be managed with collagen membranes, fibrin tissue sealants, or PRP gel. Large perforations may occur in patients with thin or friable sinus linings. These are challenging to manage, because there is often not enough membrane to support the graft. Block grafts can be inlayed in the sinus in these cases. When only a particulate graft is planned, however, surgery usually has to be aborted (unless a membrane can be used to isolate the particulate graft) and carried out after regeneration of the sinus membrane, typically 3 to 4 months later.

Oroantral fistula, chronic sinusitis, and graft infection can complicate this procedure, necessitating removal of the graft and debridement of the sinus, sometimes with simultaneous nasal antrostomy.

Numerous clinical reports suggest that in selected situations, an indirect sinus membrane lift completed through the implant preparation site will result in successful implant osseointegration. In such situations, the created space can be filled with autogenous, allogeneic, or xenograft material. It has been suggested that with small elevations, the space may simply be allowed to fill with blood with the implant acting to "tent" the elevated membrane.

Historically, autogenous bone grafts have been considered the gold standard in bone graft reconstruction for the subsinus graft procedure. Autogenous bone is osteogenic, osteoconductive, and osteoinductive. There are, however, numerous clinical studies to support the successful use of xenograft materials rather than autogenous bone such as for sinus lift surgery. A thorough understanding of the biology of xenograft incorporation and healing associated with this type of graft is required. The combined use of xenograft and the patient's autogenous bone harvested from intraoral sites may arguably provide the ideal combination of grafting with less surgical morbidity.

## Tent pole procedure

The severely resorbed mandible with less than 4 to 6 mm of residual bone may be prosthetically restored with implants using the tent pole procedure. An external incision is made in the submental region, and the entire mucoperiosteum is elevated from the mandible through this extraoral approach. Implants are placed into the thin basal bone in the best possible position without perforating the oral mucosa. Cancellous bone graft is harvested from the iliac crest, and the space created by tent pole effect of the implants that now support the elevated mucoperiosteum is packed with this graft. After at least a 6-month graft-healing period, the transoral abutments are placed.

This is a complex surgical procedure and may be complicated by mandibular or mental nerve injury; there is also the potential for mandibular fracture. A secondary intraoral vestibuloplasty may be required. This procedure has been shown to be very promising, and it does allow placement of an implant-supported overdenture for patients who have this severe anatomic resorption and who would otherwise not be able to tolerate a conventional denture (Fig 7-16).

## Distraction osteogenesis

Distraction osteogenesis (DO) is a biologic process of new bone formation between the surfaces of bone segments that are gradually separated by incremental traction. Initially applied to lengthening of leg bones in orthopedic surgery by Gavril Iliazarov, the principle of DO has been increasingly applied to maxillofacial surgery. Unlike other site enhancement strategies, DO has the potential to create much larger augmentations and also simultaneously generate new overlying soft tissue (Fig 7-17).

There are five phases in the DO process: osteotomy, latency, distraction, consolidation, and remodeling.

***Osteotomy*** The affected bone is divided into two segments, triggering the bone repair process, and a callus (bone osteoid)

**Fig 7-15** Subsinus-lift bone graft. *(a)* Lateral osteotomy and elevation of the sinus mucosa. The buccal plate may be infractured to form the roof of the graft site. *(b)* Autogenous graft is packed into the subsinus donor site.

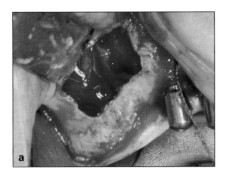
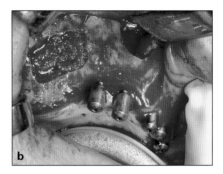

TABLE 7-2 MAXILLARY SINUS GRAFT MODIFICATIONS

| Parameter | Modification | Notes |
|---|---|---|
| Incision design | Crestal, palatal, or buccal | Crestal most versatile |
| Approach | Lateral maxillary | Most common and versatile |
| | Crestal | No advantage |
| | Osteotome technique | Augmentations of 2 to 4 mm |
| Sequencing | At time of extraction | Membrane more prone to tears<br>Roots in sinus floor |
| | With immediate implant placement | Need 4 to 5 mm of available bone to provide initial implant stability<br>Protect implants from loading during healing |
| | With delayed implant placement | If less than 4 mm of available bone or poor bone quality<br>Needs simultaneous onlay graft |
| Graft material | Autogenous bone | Gold standard with quickest healing<br>Requires second surgery<br>Maxillary tuberosity a convenient site<br>Particulate more popular than block graft and has higher success rate |
| | Allogeneic and xenogeneic bone | Convenient<br>Most work well although they require longer healing times<br>Exception: freeze-dried demineralized bone—evidence emerging suggesting results are equally good even without autogenous bone |
| Use of membranes | Lateral window coverage | Generally considered unnecessary |
| | For management of membrane tears | Resorbable membranes useful for small to medium tears<br>Helps contain particulate material |
| Other considerations | PRP | May enhance healing time and bone quality<br>Convenient consolidation of particulate material<br>Can seal membrane tears |
| | Recombinant human BMP-2 | Early though promising results<br>Very expensive |
| | Osteogenic protein | Early in the process of development |

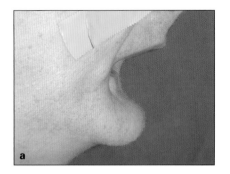

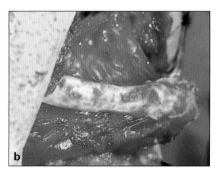

**Fig 7-16** Tent pole procedure. *(a)* Lateral view of the patient. *(b)* Exposure of the severely atrophic mandible via submental incision and without exposure of the oral mucosa. *(c)* Implants placed in residual bone. *(d)* Cancellous bone from the iliac crest covering all exposed areas of the implants.

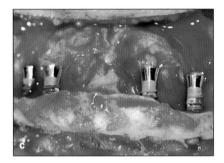

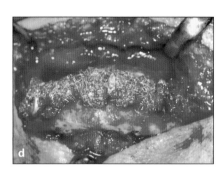

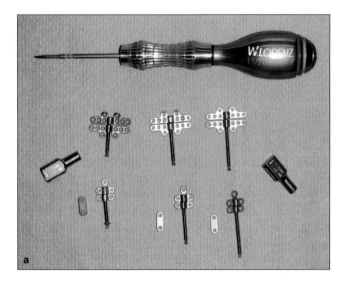

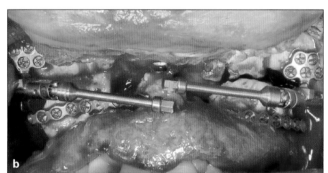

**Fig 7-17** *(a)* Different sizes of intraoral DO device (Lorenz). *(b)* Distraction appliance (KLS Martin) placed across a maxillary osteotomy site (view of the anterior maxillary midline: gingival margin of maxillary teeth at bottom; upper lip at top).

is formed. Distraction appliances are placed at this time but not activated.

***Latency phase*** Time is allowed for reparative callus to form and the bony segments and soft tissue flaps to revascularize, usually 5 to 7 days.

***Distraction phase*** Traction forces from activation of the distraction appliance gradually separate the bony segments, stretching the reparative callus and imparting a microenvironmental change at the cellular level, which has a growth-stimulating effect. New bone and soft tissue form as a result. The optimum velocity for distraction seems to be 0.5 to 1.0 mm per day, usually with slight overcorrection.

**Consolidation phase**    The distraction appliance is left in place, and the site is not functionally loaded following completion of the distraction phase. This is the time required for mineralization of the distraction regenerate. Clinically this time may extend up to 3 months, although in the case of implant surgery the time-line has been shortened by many researchers, so that implants are sometimes placed in osteoid, even before mineralization.

**Remodeling phase**    The site is functionally loaded, and the new bone progressively matures, becoming increasingly more densely calcified. It takes a year or more for the new bone to look comparable to preexisting bone.

Proponents of DO favor this technique over bone grafting and GBR because it avoids donor site surgery and graft disease transmission. It may accelerate treatment schedules and will generate new mucoperiosteum and gingiva as well as bone. Several miniaturized distraction devices have been developed, supporting the viability of DO as an alternative strategy for implant site preparation. Hybrid devices, known as *distraction implants*, have intriguing possibilities because the distraction appliance is converted to the definitive implant after the consolidation phase, simplifying treatment protocols to one surgical procedure. Studies have shown implant osseointegration to occur in both the transport segment and the regenerate during the consolidation phase. DO may indeed be the most predictable technique for vertical augmentation, although it does require a committed patient who understands the procedure and is willing to work with the appliance. These appliances are expensive, and some are cumbersome for both the surgeon and the patient. The palatal and lingual pedicles can deflect the transport segment in vertical augmentation cases, making control of the distraction vector challenging. Careful alignment and rigid fixation of extraosseous distraction appliances and appropriate direction of the osteotomy cuts are critical for success. The technique is contraindicated in patients with severe atrophy because there is not adequate existing bone available for appliance fixation. Adequate bone is also needed for safe performance of the osteotomy, avoiding vital structures such as the inferior alveolar nerve and the maxillary sinus.

Alveolar ridge augmentation achieved with DO is usually limited to one dimension only; however, multidimensional augmentations using newer angled distraction appliances have been reported. These are advanced techniques, often requiring manipulation of the distraction appliance and preoperative practice activation of the device on a stereolithic model of the patient to ensure accurate movement of the transport segment. Alveolar ridges requiring vertical and horizontal augmentation will require DO with secondary onlay grafting. Alternatively, multidimensional augmentations are probably best managed with onlay bone grafting or GBR techniques.

# Alternatives to Bone Grafting

Sophisticated reconstructive procedures have permitted the implant option to be extended to all areas of the maxilla and mandible in those patients to whom, in the early days of osseointegration, implant therapy could not have been offered. Recently, the development of new technologies, including implant modifications, has enabled graftless implant treatment in sites with deficient bone volume. These techniques include the use of short implants, the placement of conventional implants in a tilted fashion to avoid the maxillary sinus and/or the mental foramen, the zygomatic implant, and inferior alveolar nerve lateralization.

## Short implants

The use of short implants (from 6 to 9 mm in length) clearly eliminates the need for vertical augmentation in selected clinical situations. Short implants may be used in areas of ridge resorption where as little as 6 mm of vertical bone height remains, provided there remains adequate bone width.

The surgical protocol for short implants is similar to that for longer implants. Given the close proximity to adjacent anatomic structures, such as the inferior alveolar nerve or the maxillary sinus, caution must be exercised in preparing the osteotomy sites. Vertical overdrilling in the case of limited bone height in the posterior mandible may result in trauma to the inferior alveolar nerve and significant sensory abnormalities. In the case of the maxilla, penetration of the maxillary sinus or nasal floor usually results in minimal adverse sequelae.

In the past, the predominant rationale for using long implants centered on the belief that a longer implant resulted in better outcomes. Implant-loading studies, however, reveal that bone stress is concentrated mainly at the crestal region and that maximum bone stress is independent of implant length or bicortical anchorage. Implant-related stress increases somewhat with increased implant length and bicortical anchorage. Despite loading studies, however, higher failures rates have been noted with short implants. It has been postulated that this may be due to poor bone density, because these implants are more commonly used in the posterior maxilla and mandible, where there is usually a poor crown-root ratio and resultant increased bite forces. However, if parafunction is controlled and occlusion is optimized with favorable load distribution and force orientation, greater success rates, comparable to those attained by longer implants, have been reported. These goals may be achieved by altering the prosthetic design of restorations to eliminate lateral contacts on excursive movements and eliminate cantilevers. The

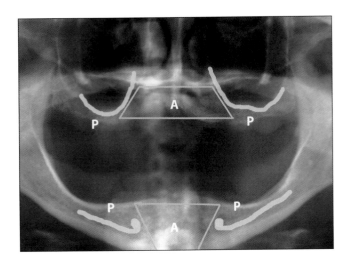

**Fig 7-18** Panoramic radiograph demonstrating zones A and P.

number of implants and the implant surface characteristics, as well as splinting of implants, may also have a positive impact on treatment outcomes with short implants.

## Tilted implants

The severely resorbed maxilla and mandible may be divided into zone A, the region anterior to the maxillary sinus or mental foramen, and zone P, the area posterior to these structures (Fig 7-18).

If bone in zone A is adequate for implants, but there is inadequate bone in zone P, graftless rehabilitation strategies enable implants in zone A, whereas implants in zone P must be placed subsequent to bone graft reconstruction. Data published since 2000 on the use of tilted implants has popularized the graftless alternative of treatment planning with implant placement solely in the areas anterior to the maxillary sinuses and the mental foramina, assuming that adequate bone is present in these regions. The most posterior implants in these cases are tilted distally, parallel to the anterior wall of the maxillary sinus, to achieve maximal distal positioning of the implants. In the case of the mandible, the tilted implants are placed just anterior to the mental foramen and the anterior loop of the inferior alveolar nerve.

By restricting implant placement to zone A and using conventional implants in a tilted fashion, the surgeon avoids adjacent anatomic structures and makes bone grafting in the posterior zones unnecessary. Tilting of an implant also allows its head to be positioned more posteriorly than otherwise possible if the implant were placed in a conventional axial fashion. Reported advantages include the need for a shorter cantilever; the use of longer implants, which may result in enhanced pri-

mary stability, particularly important if immediate loading is planned; and the avoidance of bone grafting.

Surgically, placement of tilted implants in the maxilla typically requires visualization of the anterior wall of the sinus. A small opening is made in the maxillary sinus, allowing the surgeon to identify the position and slant of the anterior wall of the sinus. The implant is then placed in a tilted fashion parallel and just adjacent to the anterior wall of the sinus. The use of a computer implant-planning program and fabrication of a custom surgical template, however, allows for a flapless surgical protocol. The angle of placement may be up to but should not exceed 45 degrees.

In mandibular cases, the mental foramen must be identified and the extent of the anterior loop respected to enable appropriate and safe placement of the distal implant. The risk of postoperative sensory nerve abnormality, although low, is a disadvantage of this technique. Computer-guided surgery may be performed in these cases, significantly minimizing this potential complication, assuming proper virtual anatomic planning is performed.

The use of four implants for a fixed prosthesis in both maxillary and mandibular edentulous cases has been popularized by Maló et al as the "All-on-Four" technique (Figs 7-19 and 7-20). Maló also advocates immediate loading for such cases. There is certainly evidence in the literature at present to support the need for fewer implants in the edentulous arch than in the earlier years of osseointegration. There is also evidence to support immediate loading in the appropriate circumstances. There are more published data, however, pertaining to the edentulous mandible than the edentulous maxilla. The All-on-Four technique for many clinicians has become a concept used in the maxilla, whereby two distal tilted implants are placed in con-

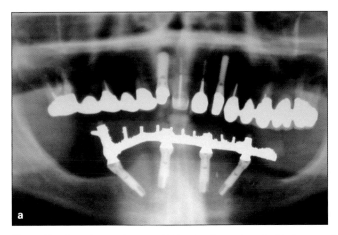

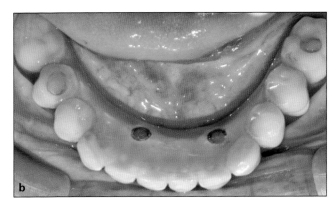

**Fig 7-19** All-on-Four technique. *(a)* Four implants placed with the two distal implants purposely tilted so that the apical area is anterior to the mental foramen and the crestal portion sits approximately in the second premolar or first molar region. *(b)* Denture supported on the four implants.

**Fig 7-20** All-on-Four technique. Maxillary implants placed so that the distal implants are skirting the anterior region of the maxillary sinus, exiting in the second premolar or first molar regions. Angled abutments on the distal implants allow for prosthetic construction.

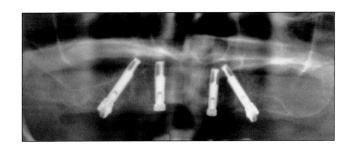

junction with as many as four anterior implants, space permitting. For many clinicians, the number of implants placed, therefore, tends to be governed by the final restorative plan, the presence of parafunctional habits, the maxillary and mandibular skeletal relationship, bone quality, whether the implants are placed in grafted sites, whether implants were previously placed in this site and failed, and any underlying patient health factors that may impart lower success rates.

## Pterygoid plate–supported implants

Tilting of implants has also been described to engage the pterygoid plates. Where there is adequate bone volume below and behind the maxillary sinus, an implant may be placed within this bone, tilted at up to 45 degrees so that the apex of the implant is through the posterior wall of the sinus, engaging the pterygoid plates for primary stability. The sinuses are bypassed and the need for grafting is eliminated. This procedure is technique sensitive; a good understanding of the anatomy is required because there are several important anatomic structures nearby, and injury may result in serious consequences.

## Zygomatic implants

The zygomatic implant was developed by Brånemark and has been in use in the atrophic maxilla since 1990. Zygomatic implants served to anchor maxillofacial prostheses in patients debilitated by cancer resections or with large clefts. The zygomatic implant, as its name implies, anchors primarily in the zygomatic bone but also in the atrophic maxillary ridge. It traverses the sinus or passes just lateral to it, depending on the morphology of the resorbed maxilla. Traditionally, it is combined with two to four conventional implants in the anterior maxilla to restore the completely edentulous patient. A patient who is partially edentulous from the canine posteriorly may also be restored with a combination of the zygomatic implant and one or two conventional axial implants.

The zygomatic implant has a prosthetic platform that is offset to the long axis by 45 degrees. This implant is available in lengths of 30.0 to 52.5 mm. Patients may be restored with either a fixed or removable prosthesis. Given the excellent initial mechanical stability of these implants due to anchorage in the zygoma, they are often immediately loaded. Conversion of the patient's complete maxillary denture to a fixed provi-

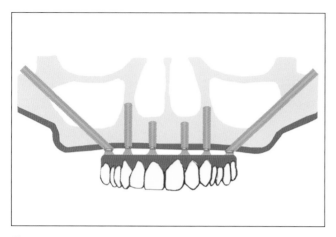

**Fig 7-21** Two zygomatic implants combined with four standard anterior implants. The zygomatic implants pass through the maxillary sinus.

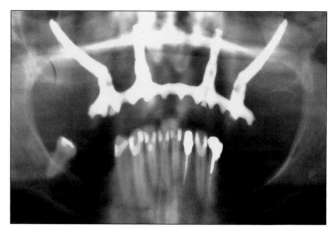

**Fig 7-22** Panoramic radiographic view of two zygomatic implants combined with two standard anterior implants. Angled abutments are placed on the zygomatic implants.

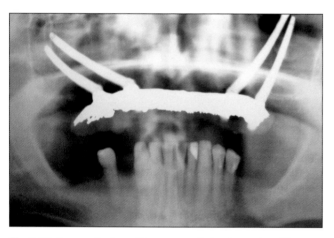

**Fig 7-23** Panoramic view of four zygomatic implants, placed because inadequate bone is available for anterior implants.

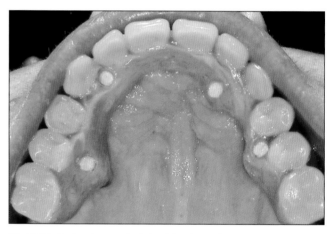

**Fig 7-24** Occlusal view of a hybrid fixed prosthesis supported on two zygomatic and two standard anterior implants.

sional prosthesis may be done the same day as the implant surgery.

Reports on the use of the zygomatic implant combined with anterior implants in delayed-loading studies in the completely edentulous patient reveal survival rates ranging from 94.2% to 100%. Interestingly, zygomatic implants have a higher survival rate than the anterior implants with which they are combined.

In cases of severe maxillary atrophy, where bone for conventional implants is inadequate in both zones A and P, two zygomatic implants may be placed bilaterally. Zygomatic implants in these cases typically exit the ridge at the lateral incisor and the second premolar or first molar sites. Fixed or removable complete-arch prostheses may be fabricated (Figs 7-21 to 7-24). At present, there is little evidence in the literature to support this technique, although it is being used in sev-

eral centers around the world with predictable, positive outcomes. The surgical technique for the zygomatic implant should be undertaken by surgeons knowledgeable about the anatomy of the region and experienced in maxillofacial surgery. Surgical exposure of the maxilla, the zygomatic buttress, and the body of the zygoma is required for implant placement. Osteotomy preparation typically includes creation of an opening into the maxillary sinus to enable clear visualization of the implant site preparation and implant placement. Traditionally, dissection of the sinus membrane off the posterior lateral wall of the sinus was recommended; however, the significance of this step is now questioned.

Despite the fact that these implants pass through the sinus, there is little reported increased risk of inflammatory reaction in this area. The development of sinusitis is uncommon. Rare

**Fig 7-25** Inferior alveolar nerve *(arrow)* isolated and retracted out of the bony canal until the implants are placed. Afterward, the nerve will be seated in the channel created and sit lateral to the implant.

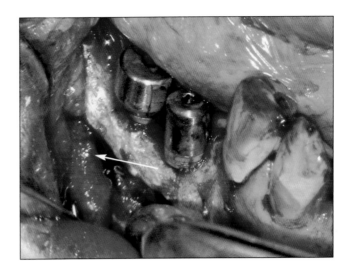

complications include penetration of the adjacent orbit and infratemporal fossa secondary to malalignment during osteotomy preparation. Meticulous attention to surgical protocol, however, prevents this occurrence.

The use of CT-guided surgical planning and execution by using specific computer-generated surgical templates is presently being developed for the use of zygoma implants.

## Inferior alveolar nerve lateralization

This technique is a treatment option that may be employed when bone height superior to the canal is inadequate for the placement of dental implants. Inferior alveolar nerve lateralization or translocation is a surgical treatment option in which the inferior alveolar nerve is moved lateral to the bony canal to allow placement of dental implants beyond this anatomic structure (Fig 7-25). With translocation, the incisive branch is transected, allowing greater mobility of the nerve. The lateral mandibular cortex overlying the area of the inferior alveolar nerve is cautiously removed, and the nerve is subsequently carefully dissected from the canal. Implants are commonly placed simultaneously with the nerve transposition and lateralization procedure.

This surgical option is technique sensitive, and the risk of permanent postoperative sensory nerve dysfunction is most likely directly related to the surgical skill of the operator. Studies support this technique, in the hands of an experienced surgeon, as being predictable with low morbidity.

# Dental Extractions in the Implant Era

## Change in surgical protocols

Implant dentistry has dramatically changed the manner in which teeth ought to be extracted. The previously accepted routine of raising a flap and removing adequate bone to expose enough of a fractured tooth or carious root to enable forceps removal is now considered excessively invasive if implant-supported prosthetics are a consideration either immediately or at some future date. To avoid bone and soft tissue loss during the extraction, hard and soft tissue preservation, or site preservation, becomes part of the surgical procedure. Wherever possible, the extraction procedure is designed to minimize loss of the labial-buccal and palatal-lingual plates.

Raising of a mucoperiosteal flap should be considered a last resort. For difficult multirooted teeth, sectioning the roots and restricting bone removal solely to the interseptal regions should be considered (Fig 7-26). This facilitates the use of a flapless technique. For challenging single-rooted teeth or retained root tips, sectioning should also be performed. In these cases, axial sectioning (along the length of the root) enables removal of the tooth in pieces with the use of fine instruments and a flapless technique. Various dental extraction devices are marketed to facilitate flapless extractions.

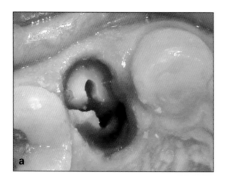 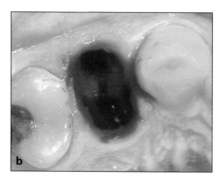

**Fig 7-26** *(a)* Sectioning of a premolar without raising a flap. *(b)* Preserved interradicular bone. An implant might be placed following extraction. It may be necessary to graft the space between the bony walls of the socket and the implant.

## Bone preservation

Alveolar bone loss occurring after dental extractions is a natural process. Some extraction sites may heal with ample bone volume maintained for implant placement, even if implant surgery occurs years later. It is difficult to predict which sites will heal in this manner. It does appear, however, that those sockets with thick labial or buccal plates and completely intact bony walls are more resistant to the rapid bone loss occasionally seen in the early postextraction period. Some surgeons consider grafting sockets with thin labial plates even if all bony walls are intact. This is particularly important in the anterior esthetic zone to help maintain the preextraction bony architecture, which ultimately affects the soft tissue contours. Socket grafting may be done with a xenogeneic, allogeneic, or alloplastic material. Some surgeons prefer to isolate the grafted extraction site with a resorbable membrane. While the required graft-healing period prior to implant placement will depend on the material used, the most predictable results will occur with a longer, rather than a shorter, graft healing time.

## Immediate implant placement

With careful planning, implant placement may be done immediately at the time of dental extraction. One of several important requirements for a successful result is initial implant stability; adequate bone must be engaged by the implant. The residual extraction site anatomy will commonly support immediate implant placement in the incisor, canine, and premolar regions, whereas the configuration of multirooted dental sockets and the surrounding local anatomy often prevents immediate implant placement at these sites.

Immediate implant placement is more challenging because the osteotomy preparation is usually placed along a different path than that of the extraction socket (Fig 7-27). In the esthetic zone, to place the implant in the appropriate three-dimensional

position, the osteotomy must be initiated on the palatal socket wall. If the osteotomy is mistakenly prepared in accordance with the actual socket axis, apical perforation will occur and, more importantly, the implant will be positioned too far labially. This labial positioning will result in a compromised esthetic outcome.

Also with immediate implant placement in extraction sites, a discrepancy between the diameter of the implant and the bony socket may be encountered; a gap is present between the socket wall and the implant. Reports are variable with regard to the need to fill these gaps with a bone graft. While there are no good clinical studies, there are many clinical reports supporting a recommendation that bone grafting of these sites is reasonable if the gaps are greater than 2 mm.

Implants immediately placed in extraction sites are often considered for immediate loading; provisional restorations that are out of occlusion are placed. The rationale for immediate loading, particularly in the esthetic zone, is to help preserve and sculpt the soft tissues to optimize esthetics. Immediate implant placement may be ideal because it eliminates the need for a second surgery. Prior consideration must be directed to the status of both the hard and soft tissues of the site; appropriate case selection is important for successful outcomes.

If the hard and soft tissues are significantly compromised, a more predictable outcome will result in the hands of most surgeons if the site is grafted primarily, followed by secondary implant placement. If the bony anatomy is favorable, but the overlying soft tissues require augmentation, the surgeon may elect to place an implant immediately and combine it with connective tissue grafting.

Contraindications to immediate implant placement include inability to achieve implant stability, localized pathology, severe hard and soft tissue defects, active periodontal disease, and acute infection. There is a lack of consensus as to the appropriateness of placing an implant in an extraction site with evidence of a chronic periapical lesion that has resulted in relatively small apical bony defects.

**Fig 7-27** Immediate implant placement following extraction of a central incisor. The implant was placed precisely as directed by the implant placement guide; however, the apical half of the implant protruded through a labial concavity. This required simultaneous autogenous and xenograft procedures. Immediate implants can create challenging surgical situations. Note that the trapezoidal flap was designed to spare the adjacent interdental papillae.

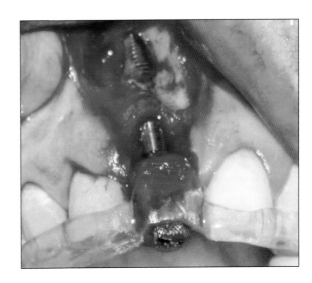

## Immediate or early function

It has been shown that osseointegration will predictably occur when implants are placed with a single-stage protocol, including immediately postextraction, with success rates similar to those obtained with the staged technique, provided that proper implant surgery approaches are followed. The desire to simplify the patient experience has led to faster loading schedules. Accelerated approaches have become possible because of changes in implant surface topography and chemical treatments, leading to more rapid bone-implant ingrowth.

Numerous studies have thus far concluded that early loading itself is not a contraindication to successful osseointegration. Rather, success is mediated by the ability to offer and maintain a load that prevents extensive micromotion at the bone-implant interface. Implant stability has been followed in some studies using resonance frequency analysis. Sequential measurements carried out over time following implant placement and loading have increased the understanding of how implant stability varies with bone healing and remodeling in the first several weeks following implantation. One-stage surgery with immediate or early implant loading in the edentulous mandible is today regarded as a routine option. Immediate loading in the edentulous maxilla as well as in partial edentulism and single-tooth cases is also more extensively reported, although the number of randomized prospective studies is still small. Some nonrandomized, prospective studies demonstrate near perfect success rates and maintenance of normal bone levels.

The advantages of accelerated-loading protocols include:

- Completion with a single surgical procedure
- Reduced prosthodontic time
- Immediate function for the patient with a secure prosthesis (provisional or final)
- Improved quality of life for the patient
- Reduced costs
- Potential to better preserve hard and soft tissue volume

Implant-loading protocols can be classified as:

- Immediate: The transitional or definitive prosthesis is attached at time of implant surgery.
- Early: The prosthesis is attached within 1 to 2 weeks.
- Delayed: There is a traditional healing time of 3 to 6 months, with single- or two-stage surgery.

Most surgical protocols call for insertion torques surpassing 30 or 35 N/cm, implant lengths greater than 10 mm, and implant widths of 3.75 mm, provided there is demonstrated excellent primary stability, before immediate prosthesis placement can be utilized. However, it is becoming more common to offer immediate loading with narrower implants. Some investigators have also used resonance frequency analysis at insertion to further measure stability, requiring a minimum implant stability quotient of 60, or a total of 200 for four implants. Protocols have been tested using four, six, or more implants, as well as distally angled implants. Implant osteotomy preparation strategies have been modified in softer bone to optimize initial mechanical stability. Techniques have included underpreparation of the osteotomy, drilling to partial depth with the last bur, minimal or no countersinking, bicortical stabilization, and the use of tapered or self-tapping implants. Such accelerated procedures are technique sensitive and are best offered by surgeons experienced in managing all aspects of implant surgery protocols.

Prosthetic principles used to enhance success in immediate-loading situations include cross-arch stabilization for complete-arch prostheses and diminished or no load for multiple- and single-tooth cases. Cantilevers are kept short; the most anterior

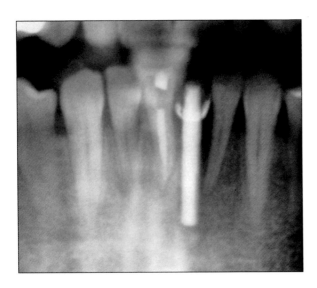

**Fig 7-28** Narrow, single-piece implant and abutment hybrid (3-mm Nobeldirect, Nobel Biocare).

and most distal implants do the work of resisting cantilever load, while the number of interposed implants provides little increased effect.

The immediate-loading principle has been combined with flapless surgery and computer-guided planning and surgical template fabrication for partial- and complete-arch cases.

## Implant-abutment hybrids

Several implant products incorporate the intraosseous screw and the prosthetic abutment as one piece (Fig 7-28). These are designed for immediate loading with a transitional prosthesis when initial stability has been achieved in good-quality bone. These abutments can be modified with a special titanium-cutting bur when necessary, although precise placement of the implant may obviate the need for this. One version of these implants has a scalloped margin mimicking the cemento-enamel junction of a tooth and may be useful for preserving bone in the esthetic zone when adjacent implants are placed.

The single-piece implant offers extra strength at the implant-abutment junction, which allows for the fabrication of very narrow 3-mm-diameter implants, in addition to larger diameter implants. The narrow implants are typically used for mandibular incisors and maxillary lateral incisors where the interradicular space or labiolingual (labiopalatal) thickness is limited. There should be 13 to 15 mm of vertical bone height. Typically, the implants are loaded with transitional crowns the day of surgery or the next day, and successful attachment of the definitive prosthesis follows 4 to 6 months later.

These implants may offer a good alternative for management of these challenging anatomic situations. Clinical results

are promising, but long-term prospective studies are pending. The one-piece implant cannot be submerged in poor-quality bone and therefore cannot be used when this type of bone prevails.

## Provisional implants

Several manufacturers offer 1.5-mm-diameter single-piece implants that are meant to be placed provisionally with the aim to stabilize transitional prostheses. They are narrow enough to place in the most confined spaces. These provisional implants require 13.0 to 15.0 mm of vertical bone. Reported favorable clinical experience includes stabilization of transitional fixed partial dentures and stabilization of complete dentures placed over arches that have been extensively grafted, aiming to prevent compressive loading of the graft and mucosal incisions. These provisional implants may loosen over time; however, this does not have a detrimental effect on the overall treatment plan. There are reports that these implants have actually osseointegrated. In these cases the abutment was cut off and the intraosseous portion of the screw was left submerged.

## SOFT TISSUE MANAGEMENT

Soft tissue management will be covered in great depth in chapter 8. However, it is germane to include soft tissue management in any discussion on surgical protocols, bone regeneration, and osseointegration. The implant surgeon must recognize the biologic similarities and differences between the healthy dentogingival junction and the tissues that make up the implant-gingival junction. The lack of a connective tissue attachment, a hypovascular-hypocellular connective tissue zone, and a blood supply with diminished collateral connections make the peri-implant soft tissue less resilient biologically. Recent implant design modifications incorporate a textured surface at the most coronal portion of the implant, leading to claims by some manufacturers that connective tissue–implant attachments can occur with these products.

The maintenance of a healthy soft tissue barrier is equally important as successful osseointegration to the long-term success of implant-supported prostheses. A stable peri-implant environment (adequate thickness of healthy connective tissue and epithelium) provides a transmucosal seal that is resistant to bacterial irritants and has sufficient structural stability to withstand the mechanical trauma commonly encountered in the oral cavity.

Patients with a thin periodontal biotype (minimal keratinized attached gingiva, highly scalloped gingival margins, prominent root contours, and thin overlying oral soft tissues) heal less predictably and have the potential for significant soft tissue loss and recession. Incision design, restoration margin placement modification, and possible preimplant soft tissue augmentation must often be considered for these patients to optimize the predictability and stability of the treatment, especially when the esthetic zone is to be restored. Patients with thick periodontal biotypes (wide bands of attached, keratinized gingiva, flat gingival scalloping, and flat periodontal contours) resist postsurgical recession but are prone to unsightly notching if releasing incisions are made in visible areas such as the gingival margin.

Inappropriate placement of the abutment-implant interface (microgap) can violate the biologic width, resulting in hard and soft tissue recession and the potential for chronic peri-implantitis. Poor soft tissue quality and quantity can compromise the esthetic outcome and the stability of the peri-implant environment. In the past, keratinized gingival tissue in the peri-implant region was considered unnecessary to long-term implant success. A growing number of investigators empirically support the presence of attached keratinized gingiva in the peri-implant environment (minimum height of 3 mm), claiming it provides enhanced support to the junctional epithelial seal.

## Soft tissue incision and flap management

Incision placement is determined by the availability and thickness of the attached gingiva and the adequacy of the lingual and palatal tissues. Historically, buccal incisions were favored because they facilitated submergence of implants in a two-stage protocol. This technique frequently resulted in excessive scarring and loss of buccal depth. Currently, favored incisions

are crestal, splitting the attached gingiva wherever possible so that suturing occurs in tough, keratinized incision margins.

More implant procedures now are performed in a single stage with immediate placement of healing abutments or transitional prostheses. This approach facilitates the lateral displacement of the keratinized, attached gingiva, effectively widening the band of this tissue (Fig 7-29).

Plastic surgery principles are incorporated in implant surgery flap design to enhance healing and to disguise the resultant scar. Palatal or lingual incision placement, beveled incisions, broad apical bases for enhanced flap blood supply, curvilinear incisions, and placement of incision lines in the interradicular depressions help to camouflage the resultant scar. Posterior flap release with anterior advancement can increase the band of attached gingiva. In cases of adequate keratinized gingiva, the incision margins can be scalloped to accommodate healing abutments or transitional restorations and simulate the natural contours of healthy gingiva.

Preservation of the interdental papilla is crucial to good esthetic outcomes. Incisions are frequently designed to leave the papilla undisturbed to minimize the risk of its loss secondary to devascularization. Papillary regeneration is possible using small cutback incisions on the labial margin of the access flap. This creates small pedicled flaps that can be rotated interdentally to create the papilla. The ability to predictably fill the interdental space with a healthy papilla, however, varies inversely with the distance between the level of the interproximal bone and the interdental contact point.

The trend in surgery has been to minimize access incisions to improve outcomes and shorten hospital stays and recovery. Minimal access or flapless surgery for dental implant placement has become increasing popular for similar reasons. Implant surgeons using this technique must be certain that the recipient site anatomy is suitable, including the presence of adequate ridge width and the absence of imperfections that would require simultaneous grafting. Bone quality must be good, because, by definition, this technique is a single-stage surgical procedure.

Flapless implant insertion does not easily support complete submergence of the implant, a strategy employed to avoid micromotion of the implant, which could adversely affect healing in cases of soft bone. The technique involves the removal of a small, circular piece of crestal gingiva. This necessitates adequate thickness of attached keratinized gingiva in the crestal region.

A modification of this technique is used when implants are placed immediately at the time of extraction. A dependable surgical guide splint assists alignment of the implant, particularly in the esthetic zone.

Flapless (Fig 7-30) implant surgery has been reported to have a very high success rate (98% to 100%), reduced early crestal bone loss, notably diminished postoperative sequelae, and enhanced patient comfort. The preservation of crestal bone blood

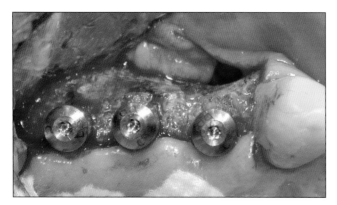

**Fig 7-29** A simple incision, scalloped and initiated more toward the palate, allows for buccal repositioning of more keratinized palatal mucosa, thereby increasing that band of peri-implant keratinized mucosa.

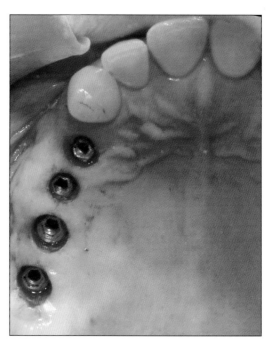

**Fig 7-30** Flapless technique to insert four maxillary implants.

supply from the soft tissue and reduction of bone manipulation are probably responsible for these results. Other observed benefits included reduced procedure time and little or no bleeding.

Modifications of the flapless approach include the U flap or palatally based island flap and its modification, the W flap. These approaches can be used for stage 1 or stage 2 surgery. They allow visualization of the palatal and interproximal bone without disruption of the labial gingiva or interdental papillae.

## Soft tissue grafting

Soft tissue grafting in sites where implant placement is anticipated is indicated where there is inadequate surrounding attached keratinized gingiva or inadequate tissue thickness. Soft tissue procedures can also be used alone for the correction of small-to-medium volume deficits and can be used to correct esthetic problems such as tissue color, surface quality, and contour. Combining soft tissue surgery with bone grafting procedures for larger deficits is also possible. Staging is often necessary to respect the potential for vascularization of the grafts, although pedicled flaps maintain their vascularity, making simultaneous procedures possible (Table 7-3).

Soft tissue healing can be guided through the use of custom abutments or provisional restorations with immediate loading when indicated by virtue of demonstrated primary stability. If immediate loading is contraindicated, a transitional interim prostheses can be fabricated to support the gingival tissues in order to guide healing in the esthetic zone. Provisional implant restorations can also be placed in a delayed approach 3 to 6 months later at stage 2 surgery. This technique requires the fabrication of custom abutments or the prefabrication, intraoperative modification, and insertion of transitional prostheses. The premise of using provisional implant restorations in the esthetic zone for 4 to 6 months prior to placing the definitive implant crowns is to allow for soft tissue maturation and guided soft tissue healing. When the plan calls for delayed insertion of a transitional prosthesis, impressions or implant registration can be carried out at the time of implant insertion so that a prefabricated prosthesis may be placed. Both appropriately contoured abutments and prefabricated provisional restorations on the implants support the peri-implant gingival cuff during healing and maturation.

### TABLE 7-3  SOFT TISSUE SURGERIES TO ENHANCE IMPLANT SITES

| Procedure | Purpose |
| --- | --- |
| *Mucoperiosteal flap procedures* | |
| Coronal advancement flap | Facilitate primary closure (especially with bone grafts) <br> Manage recession |
| Apically repositioned flap | Increase the width of attached, keratinized tissue |
| Laterally repositioned flap | Increase the width and height of the band of attached/keratinized gingiva |
| Flapless access U- and W-flap modifications | Minimal access surgery, where ridge anatomy is optimal |
| Modified palatal roll graft | Augment labial gingival contour in deficient ridges |
| Reverse cutback at incisional margins | Papillary regeneration |
| *Soft tissue grafts* | |
| Free gingival grafts | Increase band of attached/keratinized gingiva |
| Epithelialized palatal grafts | Improve tissue color, contour, and surface texture |
| Connective tissue graft | Improve tissue thickness, contour, and color (open and closed approach) <br> Correct gingival recession |
| Vascularized interpositional periosteal connective tissue graft | Vascularized, pedicled flap <br> Large augmentations, anterior maxilla <br> Good for vertical augmentations <br> Can be performed simultaneously with implant placement and bone grafts |
| Allografts | Acellular human dermal matrix* <br> Use as substitute for epithelialized palatal grafts and connective tissue grafts; avoids donor site surgery |
| *Gingival recontouring surgery* | |
| Gingivoplasty | Improve surface contour and texture using scalpel, abrasion, electrosurgery, or laser |

*AlloDerm (LifeCell).

## ACKNOWLEDGMENTS

The authors would like to thank Drs David Psutka, Lesley David, Gerald Baker, and George Sándor for the use of clinical photographs from their practices.

## RECOMMENDED READING

Aparicio C, Perales P, Rangert B. Tilted implants as an alternative to maxillary sinus grafting: A clinical, radiologic, and Periotest study. Clin Implant Dent Relat Res 2001;3:39–49.

Attard N, David L, Zarb G. Immediate loading of implants with mandibular overdentures: One year clinical results of a prospective study. Int J Prosthodont 2005;18:463–470.

Becker W, Goldstein M, Becker B, Sennerby L. Minimally invasive flapless implant surgery: A prospective multicenter study. Clin Implant Dent Relat Res 2005;7(suppl 1):21–27.

Bedrossian E, Rangert B, Stumpel L, Indresano T. Immediate function with the zygomatic implant: A graftless solution for the patient with mild to advanced atrophy of the maxilla. J Oral Maxillofac Implants 2006;21:937–942.

Block MS (ed). Implant Procedures [theme issue]. Atlas Oral Maxillofac Surg Clin North Am 2006;14:1–136.

Brånemark P-I, Gröndahl K, Ohrnell LO, et al. Zygoma fixture in the management of advanced atrophy of the maxilla: Technique and long term results. Scand J Plast Reconstr Surg Hand Surg 2004;38:70–85.

Brånemark P-I, Zarb GA, Albrektsson T (eds). Tissue-Integrated Prostheses: Osseointegration in Clinical Dentistry. Chicago: Quintessence, 1985.

Boyne PJ. The use of particulate bone grafts as barriers, eliminating the use of membranes in guided tissue regeneration. Oral Maxillofac Surg Clin North Am 2001;13:485–491.

Boyne PJ, James RA. Grafting of the maxillary sinus floor with autogenous marrow and bone. J Oral Surg 1980;38:613–616.

Campelo LD, Camara JR. Flapless implant surgery: A 10-year clinical retrospective analysis. Int J Oral Maxillofac Implants 2002;17:271–276.

das Neves FD, Fones D, Bernardes, do Prado CJ, Neto AJ. Short implants—An analysis of longitudinal studies. Int J Oral Maxillofac Implants 2006;21: 86–93.

Del Faffro M, Testori T, Francetti L, Weinsein R. Systematic review of survival rates for implants placed in the grafted maxillary sinus. Int J Periodontics Restorative Dent 2004;24:565–577.

Fiorellini JP, Nevins ML. Localized ridge augmentation/preservation. A systematic review. Ann Periodontol 2003;8:321–327.

Friberg B, Gröndahl K, Lekholm U, Brånemark P-I. Long-term follow-up of severely atrophic edentulous mandibles reconstructed with short implants. Clin Implant Dent Relat Res 2000;2:184–189.

Garg AK. Bone Biology, Harvesting, Grafting for Dental Implants: Rationale and Clinical Applications. Chicago: Quintessence, 2004.

Hammerle CH, Jung RE, Floutzis A. A systematic review of the survival of implants in bone sites augmented with barrier membranes (guided bone regeneration) in partially edentulous patients. J Clin Periodontol 2002; 29(suppl 3):226–231.

Hauschka PV, Chen TL, Mavrakos AE. Polypeptide growth factors in bone matrix. Ciba Found Symp 1988;136:207–225.

Jensen OT (ed). The Sinus Bone Graft, ed 2. Chicago: Quintessence, 2006.

Jensen OT, Pikos MA, Simion M, Vercellotti T. Bone grafting strategies for vertical alveolar augmentation. In: Miloro M (ed). Peterson's Principles of Oral and Maxillofacial Surgery, vol 1. London: Decker, 2004:223–234.

Jensen OT, Shulman LB, Block MS, Iancono VJ. Report of the Sinus Consensus Conference of 1996. Int J Oral Maxillofac Implants 1998;13(suppl 1):11–45.

Kainulaimen VT, Lindholm TC, Sándor GKS. Reconstruction of an extremely resorbed mandible by the "tent pole" procedure. Finn Dent J 2003;12:591–597.

Klongnoi B, Rupprecht S, Kessler P, et al. Lack of beneficial effects of platelet-rich plasma on sinus augmentation using a fluorohydroxyapatite or autogenous bone: An explorative study. J Clin Periodontol 2006;33:500–509.

Kushner GM (ed). Autogenous Bone Grafting [theme issue]. Atlas Oral Maxillofac Surg Clin North Am 2005;13:91–171.

Laster Z, Rachmiel A, Jensen OT. Alveolar width distraction osteogenesis for early implant placement. J Oral Maxillofac Surg 2005;63:1724–1730.

Malchiodi L, Quaranta A, D'Addona A, Scarano A, Quaranta M. Jaw reconstruction with grafted autologous bone: Early insertion of osseointegrated implants and early prosthetic loading. J Oral Maxillofac Surg 2006;64:1190–1198.

Maló P, Nobre M, Rangert B. Short implants placed one-stage in maxillae and mandibles: A retrospective clinical study with 1-9 years follow-up. Clin Implant Dent Relat Res 2007;9:15–21.

Maló P, Rangert B, Nobre M. All on 4 immediate function concept with Brånemark System implants for completely edentulous maxillae: A 1 year retrospective clinical study. Clin Implant Dent Relat Res 2005;7(suppl 1):88–94.

Marx R. Platelet rich plasma: Evidence to support its use. J Oral Maxillofac Surg 2004;62:489–496.

Misch CE. Short dental implants: A literature review and rationale for use. Dent Today 2005;24(8):64-66, 68.

Misiek D, Kent JN. In: Block MS, Kent JN (eds). Endosseous Implants for Maxillofacial Reconstruction. Philadelphia: Saunders, 1995:chap 31.

Morrison A, Chiarot M, Kirby S. Mental nerve function after inferior alveolar nerve transposition for placement of dental implants. J Can Dent Assoc 2002;68:46–50.

Noumbissi S, Lozada JL, Boyne PJ, et al. Clinical, histologic and histomophometric evaluation of mineralized solvent–dehydrated bone allograft (Puros) in maxillary human sinus grafts. J Oral Implantol 2005;31:171–179.

Oikarinen KS, Sándor GK, Kainulainen VT, Salonen-Kemppi M. Augmentation of the narrow traumatized anterior alveolar ridge to facilitate implant placement. Dent Traumatol 2003;19:19–29.

Ostman P, Hellman M, Sennerby L. Direct implant loading in the edentulous maxilla using a bone density–adapted surgical protocol and primary implant stability criteria for inclusion. Clin Implant Dent Relat Res 2005; 7(suppl 1):60–69.

Petrungaro P, Amar S. Localized ridge augmentation with allogenic bone graft blocks prior to implant placement: Case reports and histologic evaluation. Implant Dent 2005;14:139–148.

Phillips K. In: Fonseca RJ (ed). Oral and Maxillofacial Surgery. Philadelphia: Saunders, 2000:chap 11.

Pierrisnard L, Renouard F, Renault, Barquins M. Influence of implant length and bicortical anchorage on implant stress distribution. Clin Implant Dent Relat Res 2003;5:254–262.

Pikos MA. Block autografts for localized ridge augmentation. 2. The posterior mandible. Implant Dent 2000;9:67–75.

Quinn PD, Kent K, MacAfee KA. Reconstructing the atrophic mandible with inferior border grafting and implants: A preliminary report. Int J Oral Maxillofac Implants 1992;7:87–93.

Renouard F, Nisand D. Impact of implant length and diameter on survival rates. Clin Oral Implants Res 2006;17(suppl 2):35–51.

Renouard F, Nisand D. Short implants in the severely resorbed maxilla: A 2-year retrospective clinical study. Clin Implant Dent Relat Res 2005;7(suppl 1):S104-S110.

Rocci A, Martignoni M, Gottlow J. Immediate loading in the maxilla using flapless surgery, implants placed in predetermined position, and prefabricated provisional restorations: A retrospective 3 year clinical study. Clin Implant Dent Relat Res 2003;5(suppl 1):29–36.

Ryser M, Block M, Mercante D. Correlation of papilla to crestal bone levels around single tooth implants in immediate or delayed crown protocols. J Oral Maxillofac Surg 2005;63:1184–1195.

Samchukov ML, Cope J, Cherkashin A. Craniofacial Distraction Osteogenesis. St Louis: Mosby, 2001.

Sándor G. The Minimization of Morbidity in Cranio-Maxillofacial Osseous Reconstruction. Bone Graft Harvesting and Coral-Derived Granules As a Bone Graft Substitute [thesis]. Oulu, Finland: University of Oulu, 2003.

Sclar A. Soft Tissue and Esthetic Considerations in Implant Therapy. Chicago: Quintessence, 2003:197–199.

Spagnoli DB, Gollehon SG, Misiek DJ. Preprosthetic and reconstructive surgery. In: Miloro M (ed). Peterson's Principles of Oral and Maxillofacial Surgery, vol 1. London: Decker, 2004:157–188.

Tatum H. Maxillary and sinus implant reconstructions. Dent Clin North Am 1986;30:207–229.

Tawil G, Aboujaoude N, Younan R. Influence of prosthetic parameters on the survival and complication rates of short implants. Int J Oral Maxillofac Implants 2006;21:275–282.

Tawil G, Younan R. Clinical evaluation of short, machined-surface implants followed for 12–92 months. Int J Oral Maxillofac Implants 2003;18:894–901.

Vanden Bogaerde L, Rangert B, Wendelhag I. Immediate/early function of Brånemark System Tiunite implants in fresh extraction sockets in maxillae and posterior mandibles: An 18 month prospective clinical study. Clin Implant Dent Relat Res 2005;7(suppl 1):121–130.

Watzek G. Implants in Qualitatively Compromised Bone. Chicago: Quintessence, 2004.

# SOFT TISSUE ESTHETIC CONSIDERATIONS

DENNIS P. TARNOW | SANG-CHOON CHO | GEORGE A. ZARB

The health and esthetic appearance of peri-implant soft tissues are mutually dependent. Favorable long-term outcomes of both are influenced by the required synergy of several factors, namely a better understanding of wound-healing predictability, newer biomaterials, and refinement of surgical techniques. The routine clinical objective is to replicate and maintain normative esthetic parameters that reflect optimal tissue health and morphology around natural teeth. This objective is particularly relevant in the anterior or esthetic zone of the mouth and should be reconciled with each patient's circumoral activity (Fig 8-1).

This chapter discusses treatment protocols that are most likely to yield efficacious and effective long-term outcomes in the management of peri-implant morphologic tissue compromise. The ultimate objectives are an esthetically acceptable result and predictable achievement of two key determinants in treatment planning: the host bone site with its overlying soft tissue and its relationship to the interdental papilla.

## MANAGEMENT OF THE HOST BONE SITE

Surgical implant placement must be guided by the overall esthetic requirements of the definitive restoration. This strategy demands a routine three-dimensional analysis of the proposed implant site that reconciles these features in the context of an individual's circumoral activity:

- Clinical assessment and diagnostic cast analysis to provide information on mesiodistal, faciolingual, and apicocoronal dimensions
- Imaging evaluation (see chapter 6)

All too frequently, the cause of the dental absence—congenital condition, trauma, periodontal disease, failed endodontic treatment—results in different degrees of time-dependent morphologic distortion and reduction of the planned host site for the implant (Fig 8-2). Consequently, the site often needs improvement to ensure both predictable osseous support for the implant and esthetic soft tissue surroundings.

### Mesiodistal dimensions

The width of the space may have an impact on the surgical management decision. A narrow space (usually one missing tooth) is unlikely to be accompanied by a challenging reduction in vertical bone height unless the tooth was lost because of a traumatic incident with accompanying avulsion of bone or an advanced localized infective process. This stability occurs because the proximity of two healthy periodontal ligament areas adjacent to the edentulous space appears to preclude much of a ridge reduction process. The challenge in such cases is far more likely to be in the faciolingual dimension, and a narrow implant, which will have somewhat reduced optimal physical properties, usually meets the challenge in patients with a low smile line (Fig 8-3a). Otherwise, buccal grafting will be needed either before or during implant placement. The resultant interproximal papilla tends to readily assume normal proportions (Fig 8-3b).

A wide space (two or more missing teeth), on the other hand, is frequently accompanied by a time-dependent and variable vertical reduction in residual ridge height. Irrespective of the number of implants placed to support a planned fixed prosthesis, bony support for the interproximal papillae is frequently insufficient. In these situations, a mix of gingival and bony surgical strategies have to be applied to provide respect-

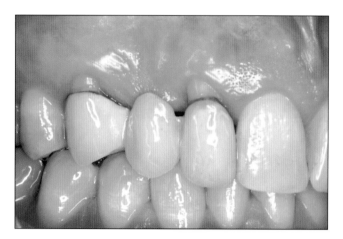

**Fig 8-1** Subtle but frequently profound management difficulties may confront the dentist, particularly when a patient's generous smile line accentuates tissue deficits.

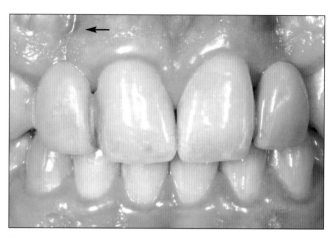

**Fig 8-2** Different degrees of time-dependent morphologic distortion and reduction of the planned host site for the implant may occur, depending on the cause of the dental absence. *(arrow)* Depression of the gingiva at the site of the maxillary right lateral incisor.

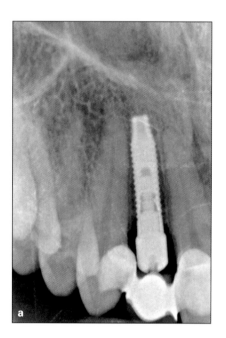

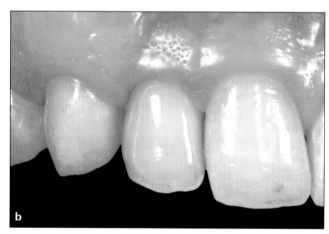

**Fig 8-3** *(a)* A narrow implant with somewhat reduced optimal physical properties has been placed in a site of limited faciolingual and mesiodistal dimension. *(b)* Interproximal papilla is obtained after buccal grafting in the area of the lateral incisor.

able esthetic results. Alternatively, a single implant and an adjacent pontic (Fig 8-4) may be the answer rather than two adjacent implants, except when two central incisors are missing.

## Faciolingual dimensions

Without question, the worst place to position an implant is too far facially. The implant should not be angled anywhere toward the labial surface. Whenever this happens, there will be great difficulty in keeping the labial tissue from migrating coronally when the new restoration is placed. The ideal placement is either at the incisal edge, if the definitive restoration will be cement retained, or slightly lingual to that (toward the cingulum area) for screw-retained restorations (Fig 8-5). If a screw-retained crown is used and the implant is placed more palatally, then the facial eminence can be created by using the crown to contour the crevice and support the buccal free gingiva.

**Fig 8-4** A single implant has been placed in the area of the maxillary right canine, and an adjacent pontic on the lateral incisor has been cantilevered over the implant on the canine to provide acceptable esthetic results.

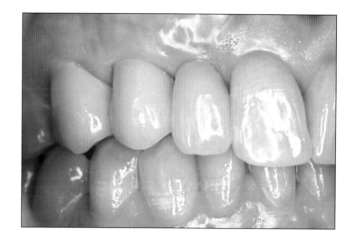

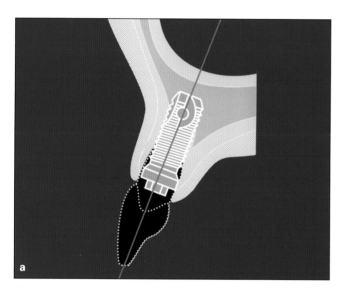

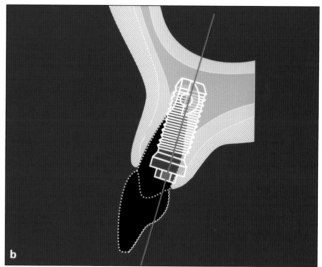

**Fig 8-5** Faciolingual angulation of implant placement. (a) Only a cement-retained restoration can be placed if the implant was placed toward the incisal edge. (b) The restoration can be screw or cement retained if the implant was placed at the cingulum.

Ideally, the implant should be placed 3.0 mm apical to the gingival margins of the proximal teeth to facilitate esthetic integration (Fig 8-6). This positioning will allow adequate space for a smooth emergence profile of the crown. If the implant placement is too shallow, and particularly if the implant is placed toward the palate, there will not be enough room to make a smooth transition in the contour of the restoration. Wherever possible, ridge lap restorations should be avoided. This design may lead to soft tissue management problems for

the patient and, without impeccable home care, to unsatisfactory long-term outcomes.

A residual ridge area with a minimal deformity that possesses a sufficient quantity of bone to allow proper implant positioning can be corrected either prior to or at the time of stage 1 surgery with a connective tissue graft. Soft tissue management at stage 2 surgery will aid in creating the appropriate tissue shape or volume in interimplant and intertooth situations. Repositioning of the tissue may be necessary to create

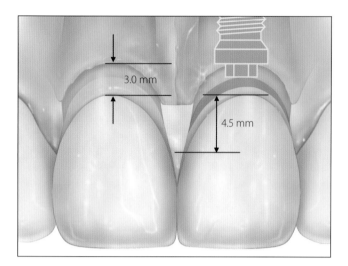

**Fig 8-6** The implant should be placed at least 3.0 mm apical to the mid-facial gingival margins of the proximal teeth to aid in esthetic integration.

the appropriate dimension of keratinized tissue and align the mucogingival junction. The incision is placed slightly lingual to the center of the implant, permitting a greater bulk of tissue to be established on the facial surface.

The tissue should be incised, not punched, in an effort to conserve tissue volume. A punch should only be used when there is an adequate dimension of soft and hard tissue around the implant. In particular, an adequate amount of attached gingiva must be present for this type of uncovering, because a punch will eliminate about 4 mm of keratinized tissue that could be saved and positioned on the facial aspect of the implant if a regular incision were performed.

Attempts to position the gingival margin coronally subsequent to the healing of stage 2 surgery are fraught with potential problems. Coronally positioned flaps and soft tissue grafting on implant restorations result in deepened crevices and are not always successful because the tissue does not adhere to the restoration. This is in contrast to midfacial recession defects on natural teeth, which are easily handled by coronal flaps with or without connective grafts. The tissues will adhere to the root surface of the natural tooth, but this is not the case with an implant restoration.

Esthetic considerations have expanded the surgical scenario for implant dentistry. Placement of an implant in a ridge that has an adequate complement of soft and hard tissues requires surgical techniques that will maintain these tissues. However, when these tissues are deficient, they must be created surgically. Evaluation of the edentulous site to establish the specific type of tissue deficiency will aid in determining the surgical sequence and the number of procedures anticipated to precede

and follow stage 1 and 2 surgeries. The purpose of these additional steps is to correct, by augmentation, the bone and soft tissue components of the ridge deformity.

A ridge defect associated with mild bone loss can be managed at the time of stage 1 surgery. A membrane and autogenous or freeze-dried demineralized bone obtained from a bone bank may be employed to correct the deformity (Fig 8-7).

Soft tissue augmentation is sometimes required on the facial surface to give the appearance of a root eminence. Similarly, the proper emergence profiles of both the provisional and final restoration are contingent on the soft tissue profile in the area of the gingival margin, which may have to be developed. To achieve this, a nonresorbable alloplast, a free soft tissue autograft, or pedicle graft can be performed at stage 2 surgery.

## Apicocoronal dimensions

Whenever a substantial amount of bone is absent from the prospective implant site, the major concern is whether it is possible to obtain surgical stability and ensure osseointegration in the preferred position. In these instances, guided bone regeneration is used to create the necessary quantity of bone in the desired location. Techniques using autogenous blocks of bone and membranes with and without bone graft material, sometimes secured in place with pins or screws, have been described. These approaches can be applied to an area that has been edentulous or at the time of tooth extraction.

Correction of these types of ridge deformities can be accomplished by modern preprosthetic surgical techniques, 6 to 9

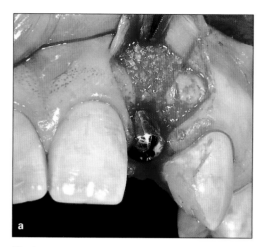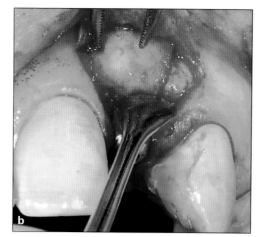

**Fig 8-7** *(a)* A ridge defect associated with mild bone loss can be managed at the time of stage 1 surgery. *(b)* A membrane may be used with autogenous or freeze-dried mineralized bone obtained from a bone bank to correct the deformity.

months prior to implant placement. Depending on the size of the initial defect and the quantity of tissue regenerated, more than one procedure may have to be performed before stage 1 surgery. At times, the bone regenerated by these procedures is not sufficient to achieve all of the desired goals in terms of housing the fixture in an adequate amount of bone and developing the necessary esthetic form. In such instances, additional osseous grafting can be performed at stage 1 surgery.

## MANAGEMENT OF THE PAPILLAE

A critical aspect in achieving appropriate soft tissue symmetry and harmony around an implant-supported restoration is preserving or creating interdental papillae.

In both stage 1 and stage 2 surgeries, incision placement is a crucial consideration. In single-tooth replacement, if the proximal teeth are less than 6.0 mm apart, the incision is made mesiodistally at the linguoproximal line angles, preserving the faciolingual dimension of the papillae and including them as part of the facial flap. However, if the teeth are more than 6.0 mm apart, the papillae are left in place, and access is achieved by the use of papillae-saving vertical incisions (Fig 8-8). This type of incision will decrease the amount of bone loss on the teeth adjacent to the implant. Exposure of the interdental bone will usually cause an average bone loss of 0.7 mm, compared to just 0.2 mm if the papillae are left intact. This may not seem like a large loss; however, because each millimeter of bone is critical to the presence or absence of the papilla, such loss should be minimized.

When papillae are missing or are insufficient to fill one or more embrasures, the clinician is confronted with a dilemma, because there are simply no predictable methods to ensure embrasure creation or enhancement. Sometimes preliminary orthodontic extrusion of teeth to help develop the papillae next to single-tooth restorations may be attempted, but this is a limited option. This topic can be discussed in three separate scenarios: the papilla between two teeth, the papilla between a tooth and an implant, and the papilla between two implants.

### Between two teeth

It has been well documented that the papilla between two teeth is heavily dependent on the distance between the contact point and the crest of the bone. If this distance is 5 mm or less, the papilla will tend to completely fill the space, and there is rarely a problem with a resultant so-called black triangle in this area.

### Between a tooth and an implant

It has also been documented that the papilla between a natural tooth and an implant is related to the level of bone on the adjacent tooth. It is the tooth and its attachment of bone and soft tissue that will support the papilla. The implant bone has little or nothing to do with this because the bone on the implant is positioned more apically than that of the tooth. For this reason, the clinician should always check the health of the periodontium on the tooth adjacent to an implant in the esthetic zone. If there is attachment loss, it may be necessary to forcibly

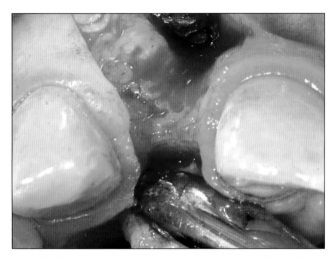

**Fig 8-8** If the teeth are more than 6.0 mm apart, the papillae are left in place, and access is achieved by the use of papillae-saving vertical incisions.

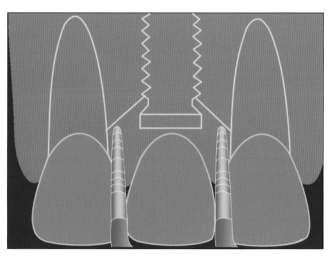

**Fig 8-9** The supracrestal biologic width on the tooth adjacent to the implant will support the interproximal papillae.

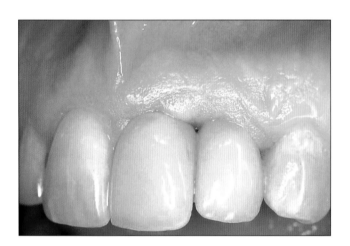

**Fig 8-10** The papilla is missing between the two adjacent implants replacing the maxillary left central and lateral incisors. The papilla at that site is shorter than the papillae next to the right central incisor and left canine.

erupt that tooth to bring the existing attachment to a more coronal position before the implant restoration is finalized.

A distance of 4.5 to 5.0 mm has been reported to be the critical distance between the contact point and the crest of the bone on the tooth for the papilla to form, a scenario similar to the one present between two natural teeth (Fig 8-9). This is why the best esthetic results are obtained with single-implant restorations placed between two periodontally healthy teeth.

## Between two implants

The main esthetic challenge for implants in the esthetic zone arises when they are adjacent to one other, especially when they are located in the central and lateral incisor positions or the lateral incisor and canine positions (Fig 8-10). In these situations, the papilla will tend to be about 2 mm shorter than it would be if two healthy teeth were still present. This is an ex-

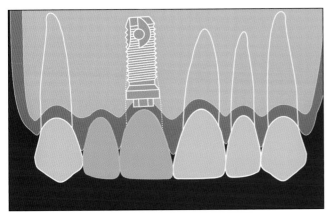

**Fig 8-11** The ideal treatment plan for central and lateral incisors that are missing unilaterally is to place one implant in the central incisor area and an ovate pontic in the lateral incisor area.

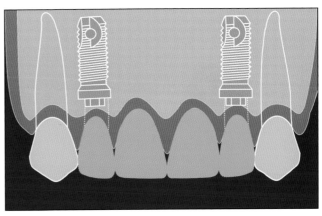

**Fig 8-12** The ideal treatment plan for two missing central incisors and two missing lateral incisors is to place two implants in the lateral incisor sites and ovate pontics between them.

tremely important consideration in treatment planning in the esthetic zone. The soft tissue attachment of the healthy tooth (the epithelial attachment and connective tissue fiber zones) is supragingival, while the resultant soft tissues in close proximity to implants are usually apical to the crestal bone. This means that the only support for an interimplant papilla is the tissue covering the crest of the interimplant peak of bone, and the level of this bone is rarely under the control of the clinician.

To date, it has not been possible to induce a supracrestal attachment of soft tissue to either implant or abutment in a manner that simulates the so-called biologic attachment described around the natural dentition. Therefore, practitioners must devise ingenious alternative management protocols in their collective efforts to simulate normative dimensions for particularly challenging deficit situations.

When two central incisors are missing and are to be replaced with two adjacent implants, a favorable esthetic outcome very frequently can be achieved. Although the papilla between these restorations will be shorter than ideal, the clinician can modify the crowns and create a broader, flatter contact. As long as the papilla still has a V shape, the appearance is usually acceptable, because it harmonizes with the midline of the face, and asymmetry is avoided.

However, a problem occurs if the two teeth are not in the center of the arch, such as a central and a lateral incisor or a lateral incisor and canine. In these situations, a resultant short papilla creates an asymmetry compared with the contralateral side. This so-called black triangle may be bothersome to the point of being esthetically unacceptable to some patients and is difficult to rectify with a simulated gingival triangle of pink porcelain to fill the space.

A possible solution is to place an implant in the central incisor area and then cantilever an ovate pontic in the lateral incisor position (Fig 8-11). The rationale is that an ovate pontic has, on average, only about 0.7 mm less height than if an adjacent tooth were present, a favorable comparison with a papilla that would on average be 2 mm shorter. Furthermore, a pontic area can always be grafted to expand the soft tissue, but if two adjacent implants are present there is simply no predictable way to graft the papilla back.

If four incisors are missing, the ideal approach would be to place the implants in the lateral incisor positions and then place two ovate pontics in the central incisor positions (Fig 8-12). This would allow the distal papillae to be supported by the canines. The clinician can then carry out soft tissue augmentation as needed to increase the soft tissues in the area between the two central incisors.

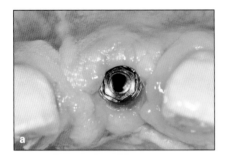

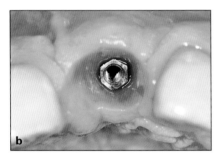

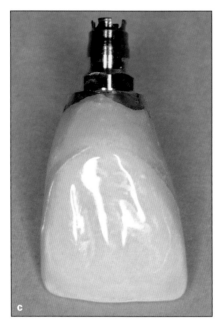

**Fig 8-13** *(a)* Healing abutments do not reflect the differences between mesiodistal and faciolingual dimensions of a natural tooth. An appropriately shaped working crevice *(b)* for the definitive restoration may be sculpted with a provisional restoration *(c)* that is prefabricated and inserted at stage 2 surgery.

## Additional Considerations

Healing abutments are available in various diameters, but they do not reflect the differences between mesiodistal and faciolingual dimensions of a natural tooth. An appropriately shaped working crevice for the final restoration may be facilitated with a provisional restoration that is prefabricated and inserted at stage 2 surgery (Fig 8-13). This is done by taking an impression at the time of implant placement. The resultant crevice appears to anticipate the shape of the final restoration and even permits incremental addition to the provisional restoration, which in turn influences the shape of the surrounding crevicular tissue via pressure that allows the tissues to adapt to their new position. This will also facilitate papillary formation until the fixed contact point is established by the provisional or final crown.

The focus of research for the future will be to give the clinician the ability to predictably achieve supracrestal attachment to either the implant or the implant-abutment combination. This will allow a better result for the interdental papillae, as discussed previously. This is also where the concept of a scalloped-top implant has come into play. The peaks of the scallop must be placed interproximally, and they must be positioned supracrestally in order to locate the biologic width in a more coronal position. Therefore, the procedure in the future will be either to scallop the implant top and position it properly or to scallop the abutment.

To keep the tissue attachment supracrestal, the abutment must not be changed. In other words, whatever abutment will be used for the final abutment is the one that should be placed as soon as the implant is exposed to the oral cavity. If the abutment is changed repeatedly the biologic width will move apically and the benefit for the papillary support will have been lost.

Many capable and experienced clinicians have recommended specific abutment designs or even so-called platform switching in their efforts to achieve better control over the final morphology of the peri-implant soft tissues. These initiatives are paralleled by commercial claims for hardware design that can induce a healed response of bone height development that ensures the creation and maintenance of optimal interproximal support for an esthetic papilla. These well-intentioned claims must be regarded as anecdotal, however, because they lack rigorous documentation, let alone compelling outcome results.

## CONCLUSION

Providing a patient with a functionally and esthetically successful implant-supported restoration frequently requires an appropriate sequencing of treatment. The professionals involved in such treatment anticipate deficiencies in the proposed host bone and soft tissue sites. The presenting morphology and contour of many partially edentulous residual ridge deformities require a staged and often variable management approach. In these instances, orthodontic movement, guided tissue regeneration to increase osseous volume, soft tissue surgery, or most reliably autologous bone grafts may be indicated as separate or combined procedures.

With careful assessment, a decision can be made as to when the required surgical correction will be most effectively performed. A well-executed and predictable osseointegrated and esthetic result can be accomplished in the shortest period of time with the fewest invasive procedures with diligent and conscientious treatment planning.

## RECOMMENDED READING

Abrahamsson I, Berglundh T, Lindhe J. The mucosal barrier following abutment dis/reconnection: An experimental study in dogs. J Clin Periodontol 1997;24:568–572.

Choquet V, Hermans M, Adriaenssens P, Daelemans P, Tarnow D, Malevez C. Clinical and radiographic evaluation of the papilla level adjacent to single-tooth dental implants. A retrospective study in the maxillary anterior region. J Periodontol 2001;72:1364–1371.

Esposito M, Ekestubbe A, Grondahl K. Radiological evaluation of marginal bone loss at tooth surfaces facing single Brånemark implants. Clin Oral Implants Res 1993;4:151–157.

Garber DA, Salama MA, Salama H. Immediate total tooth replacement. Compend Contin Educ Dent 2001;22:210–218.

Gomez-Roman G. Influence of flap design on peri-implant interproximal crestal bone loss around single-tooth implants. Int J Oral Maxillofac Implants 2001;16:61–67.

Grunder U. Stability of the mucosal; topography around single-tooth implants and adjacent teeth: 1-year results. Int J Periodontics Restorative Dent 2000;20:11–17.

Lazzara RJ, Porter SS. Platform switching: A new concept in implant dentistry for controlling postoperative crestal bone levels. Int J Periodontics Restorative Dent 2006;26:9–17.

Parel SM, Sullivan DY. Aesthetics and Osseointegration. Dallas: Taylor, 1989.

Salama H, Salama M. The role of orthodontic extrusive remodeling in the enhancement of soft and hard tissue profiles prior to implant placement: A systematic approach to the management of extraction site defects. Int J Periodontics Restorative Dent 1993;13:312–333.

Pikos MA. Facilitating implant placement with chin grafts as donor sites for maxillary bone augmentation—Part I. Dent Implantol Update 1995;6:89–92.

Tarnow D, Elian N, Fletcher P, et al. The vertical distance from the crest of bone to the height of the interproximal papilla between adjacent implants. J Periodontol 2003;74:1785–1788.

Tarnow DP, Magner AW, Fletcher P. The effect of the distance from the contact point to the crest of bone on the presence or absence of the interproximal dental papilla. J Periodontol 1992;63:995–996.

Wohrle PS. Enhanced aesthetic outcome based on biological principles: The scalloped implant. Periodontol 2000 2003;1:13–21.

# Prosthodontic Considerations

George A. Zarb | Steven E. Eckert | Clark Stanford

Loss of teeth mainly results from neglected or inadequately managed disease processes or, less frequently, trauma. The resultant outcomes are often manifested as combinations of functional and esthetic treatment challenges. Although traditional management resulted from outstanding treatment technologies, it would be wrong to assume that prosthodontic interventions per se actually treat disease processes. In fact, it could be argued that other forms of adverse change may be catalyzed by treatment, such as the varying degrees of residual ridge resorption associated with wearing complete dentures or removable partial dentures.

Additional ecologic risks are involved in management of partial edentulism: recurrent caries as well as pulpal and periodontal disease. The ingenuity of removable and fixed partial denture interventions (Figs 9-1 to 9-8) evolved to address the consequences of teeth loss, but did little to manage the com-promised intraoral ecology that necessitated intervention in the first place. These well-documented outcomes are a sober reminder of the fact that, while technology can be used to manage the sequelae of disease, it is ecologically driven biotechnology that helps control future progression of disease. Therefore, it is important to reemphasize the ever-present prosthodontic treatment dilemma: What is the ecologic price implicit in both the morphologic predicament of tooth loss and its management?

To facilitate an understanding of currently employed prosthodontic protocols for managing partial and complete edentulism, this chapter will highlight aspects of how osseointegration evolved as a clinical routine. First, however, a preliminary synthesis of relevant occlusal, esthetic, and timing-of-placement considerations will serve as a useful introduction to specific clinical situations discussed later in the chapter.

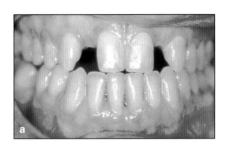
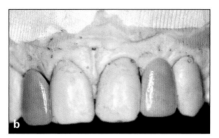
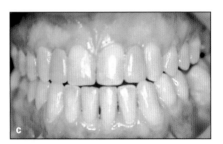
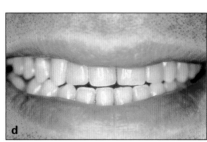

**Fig 9-1** Congenitally missing maxillary lateral incisors *(a)* have been replaced bilaterally with adhesive prostheses *(b to d)*.

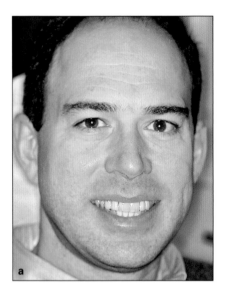
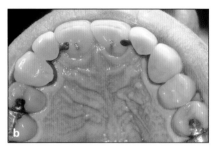

**Fig 9-2** *(a and b)* Congenitally missing maxillary lateral incisors have been replaced bilaterally with fixed cantilevered two-unit prostheses.

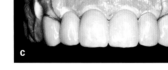
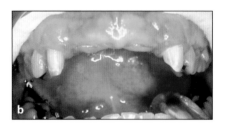
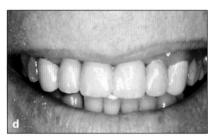

**Fig 9-3** Missing traumatically avulsed incisors *(a and b)* have been replaced with a six-unit fixed prosthesis *(c and d)*.

**Fig 9-4** *(a to d)* Complete-arch rehabilitation has been accomplished with fixed prostheses exclusively.

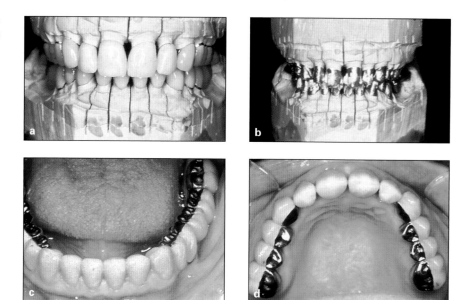

**Fig 9-5** Complete-arch rehabilitation has been accomplished with combined fixed-removable prostheses

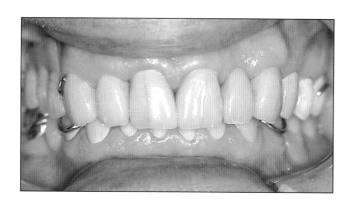

**Fig 9-6** *(a to d)* Complete-arch rehabilitation accomplished with combined fixed-removable prostheses in another patient.

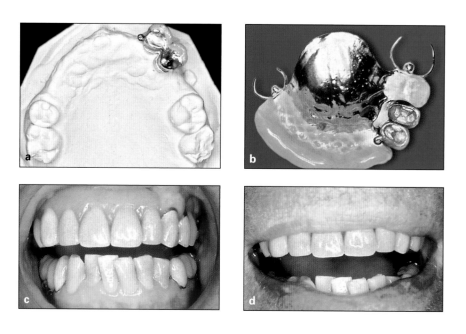

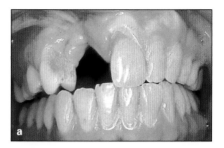

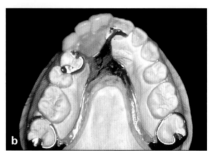

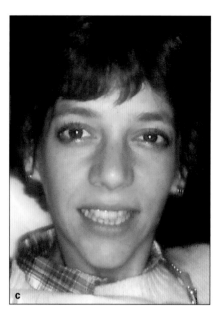

**Fig 9-7** *(a to c)* A removable prosthesis was employed to provide comprehensive functional restoration for an adult with an operated unilateral cleft lip and palate.

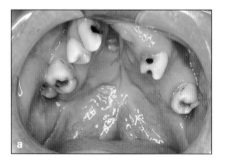

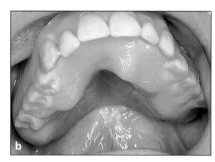

**Fig 9-8** *(a and b)* A complete maxillary overdenture was prescribed to restore function and esthetics for this surgically repaired but otherwise untreated adult cleft palate patient.

# OCCLUSAL CONSIDERATIONS

An appreciation of the role and diversity of the occlusal interface is an integral part of prosthodontic treatment. However, a clear understanding of the actual role of occlusion in health and disease has proven to be elusive because their possible link remains controversial. Consequently, attempts to reconcile treatment objectives of restoring occlusions with specific technique protocols that rely on occlusal theories, articulators, and favored restorative materials have only confused dentists. Such stylized diagnostic and treatment prescriptions are all too often advocated as "all or none" essential requirements but lack scientific validity. They also overlook the foundation for occlusal treatment in prosthodontics, namely the following tenets:

- Prosthodontics evolved from a mechanical era when biologic factors were poorly understood.
- Recent critical reviews of the discipline's core values have shifted focus to its biologic roots and the variable but significant psychosocial, functional, and esthetic implications for most patients.

- The range of normative values of anatomic (form), physiologic (function), and esthetic variations encountered should also be assessed in both time-dependent and parafunctional contexts.
- The absence of long-term outcome data from clinical interventions underscores the merits of employing normative determinants as outcome objectives when treatment plans for occlusal changes are developed. The determinants we recommend were first described by Henry Beyron almost 40 years ago (Box 9-1 and Fig 9-9).
- Occlusal design for implant-supported prostheses is an essential and integral determinant of overall treatment planning. It is a very early priority in the reconciliation of optimal force distribution to maximize axial loading and in achieving the desired esthetic result. It cannot be relegated to afterthought status as occlusal adjustment casts and articulating paper are very poor substitutes for correct design in occlusal management.

**Box 9-1** BEYRON'S DESCRIPTORS OF NORMATIVE OCCLUSIONS

- Maximum number of bilateral centric stops
- Adequate vertical dimension of occlusion
- Freedom in retrusive range of occlusal contact
- Multidimensional freedom of contact movement

These descriptors provide guidelines for obtaining treatment efficacy and effectiveness when the clinician is changing a nonphysiologic occlusion to a therapeutic occlusion:

- *Nonphysiologic occlusion*: Where signs and symptoms of abnormal function are present because of lack of adaptation in the masticatory system. It typically includes deficient or compromised dental, osseous, or neuromuscular structures. The patient may not be satisfied with function or esthetics.
- *Therapeutic occlusion*: An occlusion that has been corrected or restored to fulfill the proposed guidelines.

**Fig 9-9** The Beyron descriptors underscore the similarities between the normative relationships of a natural dentition *(a to d)* and those readily built into an artificial one, irrespective of whether the occlusion is destined to be supported by soft tissue, as in this laboratory complete denture setup *(e)*, or implants *(f)*. Note that these illustrations are two-dimensional and do not purport to demonstrate the dynamic relationships that are also an implicit part of the Beyron description.

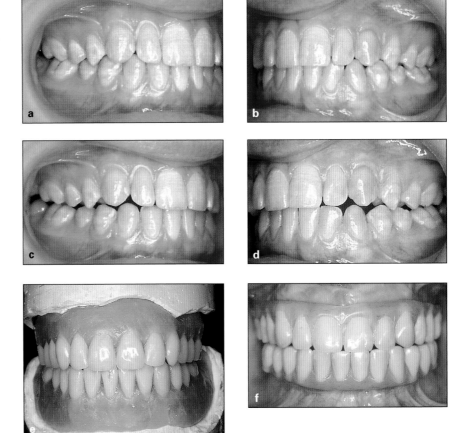

When considering the occlusion of restorations supported and retained by endosseous implants, the clinician must remember the differences between implants and natural teeth. Natural teeth are suspended in the dental alveolus by a periodontal ligament that allows slight physiologic movement in all directions. In the event of excess occlusal forces, the tooth may become mobile, exhibit excessive wear, or even fracture.

In contrast, osseointegrated implants are "ankylosed" and demonstrate virtually no mobility within the bone. When forces are excessive, the implant lacks the capacity to adapt physiologically through increased mobility. In such a situation, the result of excessive force on an implant-supported restoration could be intrusion of the opposing teeth; abrasion of the opposing teeth or restorations; fracture of restorative material on the implant-supported restoration; loosening of abutments, cement, or prosthetic retaining screws; or loss of osseointegration. The last result is hypothesized on the basis of interfacial microfractures that develop in response to adverse loading and that may continue to grow and coalesce, thereby undermining the implant's stability. Subsequent compromise of the implant's bone support and the risk of increasing mobility are presumed to be irreversible and to leave the implant vulnerable to infective processes.

Although somewhat anecdotal in nature, observations of a higher than average incidence of fracture of prosthetic materials in implant-supported restorations have been made by many clinicians. This appears to be a fairly predictable situation, because implants lack the capacity to dampen the force applied to the implant-supported restoration. Consequently, the forces are transmitted to the prosthetic material, which, in many cases, is a brittle ceramic. Although ceramic materials have high compressive strength, they are incapable of withstanding high-intensity, short-duration trauma, which seems to explain the higher fracture rate.

The lack of mobility in an osseointegrated implant can be compensated for in a number of different ways. The historic developmental approach was to permit a weak link in the restoration. Rather than creating a rigid prosthetic connection to implants, early designs used a prosthetic retaining screw that would loosen or fracture under high load. The approach eventually lost some of its popularity, and many current restorations are luted to the transmucosal abutment with den-

tal cements. This latter approach appeals to dentists because of its familiarity—a lateral move from traditional fixed prosthodontic protocols. It has also has been advocated because of the perception that modern abutments are relatively immune to mechanical complications such as screw loosening or fracture. Other clinicians are not completely convinced of the wisdom of such an approach and advocate the use of weaker provisional cements to allow retrieval of the prosthesis in the event of screw loosening.

The practice of cementing implant-based prostheses can often be at odds with the likelihood of biologic and technical failure. The literature certainly suggests that, even in the hands of experienced operators, complications occur frequently enough to concern clinicians with less experience. The virtual irretrievability of cemented prostheses is therefore an important consideration in making a decision that may compromise or eliminate the desired recovery potential of most prosthodontic designs.

Because the entire implant-abutment-prosthetic system is linked in a straight line, efforts to reduce the impact of otherwise uncontrollable occlusal forces must be considered. Any angulations of the occlusal surfaces of the restoration can create vector forces and moments of force within the implant-abutment-prosthetic system. Therefore, these moments of force can be reduced by the creation of a flatter occlusal surface. Likewise, deep grooves within the occlusal surface should be minimized to avoid foci of bolus localization or impaction, which could in turn adversely alter force transmission.

It is therefore prudent to recall Skalak's original objective that all the interdependent components of a fixed implant-supported prosthesis have immobile connections: framework to abutments to implants to bone (Fig 9-10). The achievement of such a trusslike effect precludes relative movement between prosthesis and its support and of course implant and bone, and moreover it seems to apply even if abutments are always parallel. This theoretical objective appears to be readily reached in most multiunit tooth replacement situations, but its efficacy is dependent on meticulous attention to all the components of the clinical endeavor.

Occlusal force considerations in the context of implant support are summarized in Box 9-2.

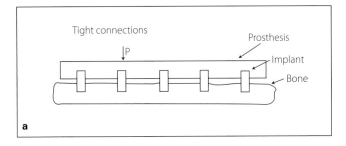

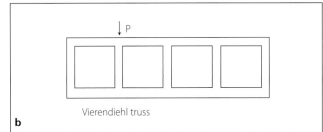

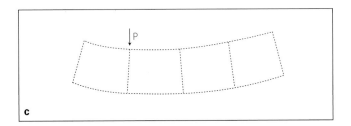

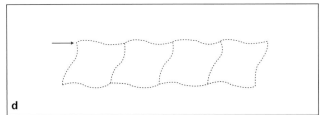

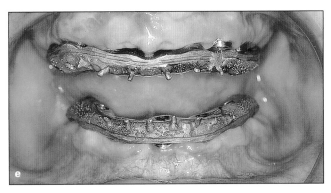

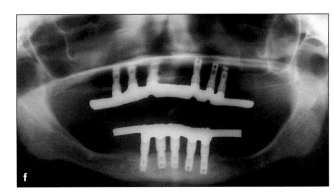

**Fig 9-10** *(a)* Skalak's schematic sketch of a fixed prosthesis connected to the bone via a tight osseointegrated connection and subjected to both vertical (P) and horizontal loads. *(b)* The effective integral structure is a Vierendiehl truss in which each joint is rigid and can carry bending movements. *(c and d)* Qualitative behavior and deflection of the combined structure under vertical and horizonal loads. *(e and f)* The original Skalak characterization of a Vierendiehl truss is similar to the immobile connections between implant components—prosthetic framework, abutments, and implants—and host bone and underscores the importance of the relative immobility of the simulated truss.

---

**Box 9-2 OCCLUSAL FORCE MANAGEMENT THAT MAY BE CONTROLLED BY THE DENTIST**

1. Whenever feasible, seek to direct occlusal forces along an implant's long axis.

2. Try to minimize tipping forces such as distal or buccal cantilevering since they may turn out to be mechanically harmful.

3. Cyclical loads may compromise the integrity of mechanical components, hence the prudence of anticipating both cyclical and sustained loads of parafunctional activity.

4. Loading of the implant's healing interface may be hazardous for that implant's osseointegrated longevity.

5. It does not appear that the choice of occlusal surface impacts the survival or longevity of implant treatment.

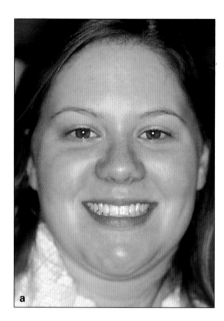

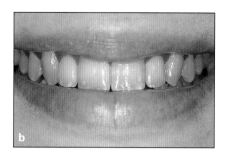

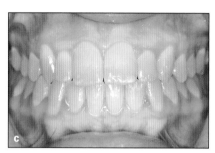

**Fig 9-11** Although clearly not a panacea or a substitute for scrupulous surgical judgment, the introduction of angulated abutments has proven to be invaluable for many clinical situations where respectable esthetic results would have otherwise been precluded. *(a to c)* Implants in the maxillary lateral incisor sites were placed with unavoidable labial angulations because of host bone morphology but were readily corrected with angulated abutments.

# Esthetic Considerations

Once they are osseointegrated, endosseous implants provide absolute retention and support for dental prostheses. Unfortunately the shape or anatomic configuration of endosseous implants differs from that of natural teeth. Additionally, endosseous implants have traditionally been fabricated from metals (primarily commercially pure titanium and alloys of titanium) that do not possess the translucent properties of natural teeth. As a result, the clinician is invariably faced with the task of compensating for the differences between the physical appearances of implant components and natural teeth.

The emergence of a prosthetic restoration from an endosseous implant inevitably differs from the way a crown emerges from the roots of a natural tooth. A variety of angulated transmucosal abutments have been designed to compensate for the difference in angulation between the crown and the implant that serves as a root analog. These transmu-

cosal abutments have minimized some of the esthetic liabilities associated with restoration of endosseous implants and permitted very respectable esthetic results (Figs 9-11 and 9-12). However, it would be naïve to presume that all unfavorably tilted implants can be recruited into an optimally esthetic treatment result.

Even the most scrupulously planned and executed implant treatment is ultimately driven by the overall challenge of achieving successful osseointegration. The mere provision of stable tooth root analogs will not routinely fulfill all the desired esthetic clinical outcomes. It remains prudent and correct to state that scrupulous planning and teamwork between surgical and prosthodontic professionals frequently succeed in providing esthetic fixed or removable prostheses. However, implants are definitely not a panacea for patients' esthetic expectations. Hence the following points must be kept in mind:

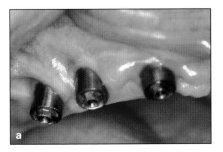 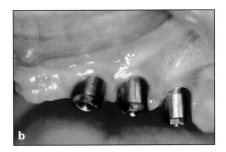 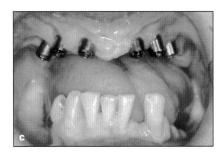

**Fig 9-12** The angulated abutments *(a to d)* used for a maxillary complete-arch prosthesis *(e and f)* ensured that a fixed solution was possible when bone morphology dictated labially angulated implant placement.

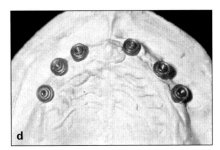

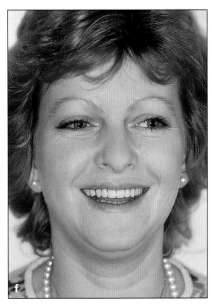

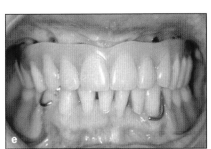

- Textbook-perfect treatment outcomes are often described in publications and presented at meetings. Although these splendid looking case histories are much admired by esthetic study clubs and similar organizations, they are often the result of increased costs and treatment times as well as multiple surgical soft tissue interventions. Moreover, these applications tend to demand exceptional surgical skills and all too often ignore the possibility of simpler and more predictable prosthetic solutions.
- So-called ideal surgically enhanced esthetics may be indeed feasible for selected situations. However, the vast majority of esthetic challenges can be readily and simply addressed through scrupulous treatment planning by the dentist and the ceramist. In overall treatment planning, absolute emphasis on the surgical intervention does not relegate the prosthetic rehabilitative aspect to an inferior role. Most challenging situations demand a trade-off approach between surgical enhancement and prosthodontics that can be readily addressed via repeated try-ins of the planned prosthesis and

the occasional fabrication of a provisional one. These special case histories are often managed as works in progress and have to be assessed over time. This strategy permits a better appreciation for both patient and tissue responses and a more likely satisfactory outcome.
- A primary esthetic objective is to compensate for the appearance of the implant (usually in short-span replacement situations) with the final restoration whenever the clinician is faced with the task of placing the implant in a poor position relative to alveolar bone and oral mucosa. In the esthetic zone, this problem is best avoided by appropriate location and development of an implant site that allows the implant to be placed with sufficient thickness of bone facial to the implant to resist bone loss and to ensure that the color of the implant or the collar on an angulated abutment does not show through the labial tissue (Fig 9-13). However, now it is frequently possible to compensate for esthetically unfavorable implant placement with ceramic or zirconium abutments.

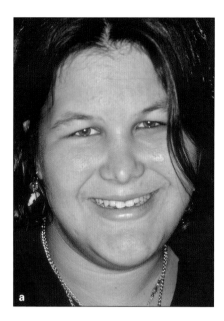

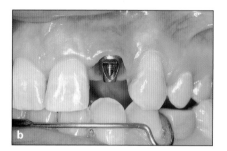

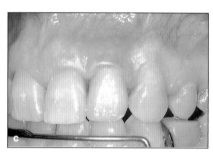

**Fig 9-13** A favorable smile line *(a)* only incompletely masks the labial gingival purplish hue *(b and c)* introduced by the underlying metal collar on the angulated abutment. This minor inconvenience is now virtually precluded by using customized nonmetallic abutments.

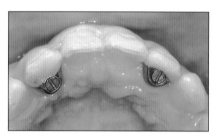

**Fig 9-14** An unsightly "show-through" of the implant's cervical metal also often can be avoided by a more palatal surgical placement of the implant in the first place.

The ability to customize abutments in combination with cemented crowns popularized the evolving approach to anterior tooth replacement, particularly single-tooth replacement. In most situations, if the sagittal morphology of the host bone site is favorable, the implant can be actually placed somewhat more palatally or lingually (Fig 9-14). The restoration can then be luted or even screw retained because there is no concern with screw emergence. However, placement of the implant too far toward the palate may result in a lack of support for the facial gingival tissue. In this rare situation, the attendant lack of cervical gingival support can only be approximated by creating a ridge lap design with the crown restoration. Although this design is feasible, it may make hygiene maintenance awkward.

## Ceramic components

Recent developments in the use of ceramic transmucosal abutments have already demonstrated a more favorable soft tissue response. The primary advantage of ceramic materials is that they are somewhat translucent and of a color that is more similar to the natural tooth. These abutments are generally coupled with all-ceramic restorations to create relatively life-like analogs of natural teeth. The long-term clinical performance of these abutments has yet to be documented in scientific studies. Consequently, clinicians are cautioned to use ceramic abutments only when necessary for esthetic reasons and to provide the patient with informed consent regarding the use of such materials.

## Soft tissue appearance

As discussed in the previous chapter, the objective of any restoration is to simulate the emergence of the natural tooth from its surrounding tissues. Adjacent teeth will serve as a guide toward the gingival emergence of an implant-supported restoration. In many instances either gingivoplasty or gingival augmentation is necessary to contour the soft tissue to simulate that of the adjacent teeth.

The position of the interdental papillae is primarily established by the relationship between crestal bones relative to the adjacent teeth. The distance from the interdental bone crest to the most incisal portion of the papilla is generally 4 to 5 mm. This dimension should be considered when an implant is placed in relatively close proximity to another implant. When two implants are adjacent to each other, the interdental (in this case, interimplant) papilla is lost. Soft tissue that mimics a papilla may continue to exist, but the height of that tissue relative to the interimplant residual alveolar crest rarely exceeds 3 mm.

# Timing-of-Placement Considerations

The timing of implant placement relative to the time of tooth extraction has received much more attention in recent years. A departure from the original staged protocol was articulated on the basis of both overall treatment convenience and the desire to preserve bone by placing an implant in a fresh extraction socket. Many authors believe that when teeth are removed and implants are placed immediately, the residual alveolar ridge does not heal with a vertical or horizontal defect. Others suggest that this relatively predictable procedure sometimes results in exposure of the endosseous implant if bone healing does not proceed according to plan. Members of the prosthodontic community have long been aware of the vagaries of postextraction bone-healing behavior and are inclined to be somewhat skeptical of the premise of predictable cervical bone levels in association with immediate implant placement. The bottom line is that bone levels following healing are not readily predictable for different sites following the different reasons that account for loss of a tooth.

Nonetheless, whenever an implant is placed immediately following tooth removal, the extraction technique is important, and every effort must be made to preserve the critical labial plate of bone; simultaneous facial bone augmentation may also be advantageous. Previous periapical infections must be thoroughly debrided to prevent contamination of the implant, and postsurgical antibiotic administration may help implant survival.

From a practical standpoint, it seems reasonable to suggest that the highest likelihood of implant survival occurs when implants are placed in well-healed alveolar bone because tooth removal does not always result in favorable healing. Yet it must be acknowledged that there is always the risk that alveolar structure will fail to return to preextraction height if tooth removal is followed by a healing period before an implant is placed.

Loss of a thin labial or buccal plate of bone following tooth extraction could also cause concern when the definitive restoration is planned. When this occurs in an area of high esthetic concern, it may become necessary to develop the implant site prior to implant placement. Numerous labial bone augmentation techniques, including allografts, alloplasts, xenografts, guided bone generation, and connective tissue grafts, have been advocated for site development. The clear choice of augmentation method may be more dependent on the practitioner's individual clinical skills than on the superiority of any specific technique (see chapter 7).

# Protocols for Edentulous Patients

Edentulism, or total periodontal ligament deficit, can now be reliably and routinely rectified with implant-supported and -retained prostheses. This extraordinary therapeutic breakthrough has now become one of the most compellingly documented modalities in prosthodontics. Some of its key features will be identified to underscore the technique's current and well-documented versatility and excellent prognoses. They also provide a starting point for the subsequent lateral protocol move to managing partial edentulism, particularly in the anterior zone.

## Prosthetic design

The initial protocol described 5 to 6 implants in the anterior zone as readily supporting 10- to 12-unit fixed prostheses. It was a prudent if slightly restrictive approach in the broader esthetic and functional context. For mechanical reasons, the protocol dictated that the length of the cantilever extension had to be limited to 15 to 20 mm in the mandible and 10 to 15 mm in the maxilla. The resultant variation on the theme of a somewhat shortened dental arch proved versatile and effective (Fig 9-15), but it was not universally applicable.

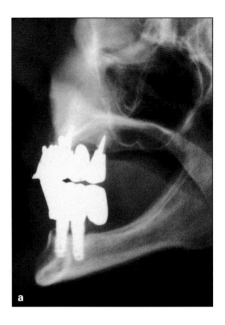

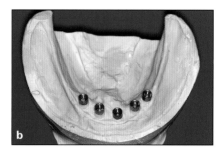

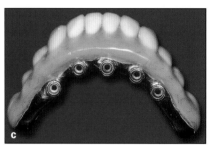

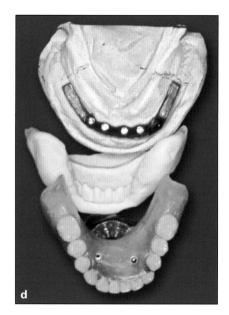

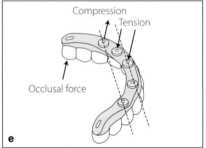

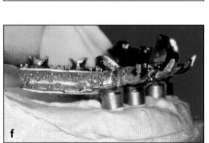

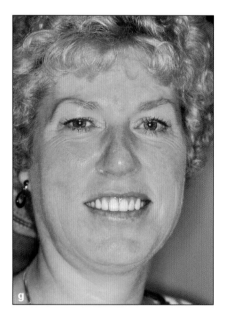

**Fig 9-15** *(a to f)* The initial developmental protocol for an implant-supported dentition for an edentulous patient reconciled implant lengths and numbers with their specific location, material strength considerations, and presumed functional dictates. Shortened dental arches were a frequent result, although the esthetic outcome was rarely compromised *(g)*.

Consequently, the 5- to 6-implant-support formula quickly expanded to 8 or more for specific situations, a feature that became even more accessible with refinements in surgical technique (such as sinus lifts) and the introduction of wide-bodied implants (Fig 9-16). Wide and generous smiles, plus a natural or restored opposing dentition, frequently demanded more prosthetic teeth and additional posterior implant support. The surgical community was readily and happily recruited for the new protocol of placement of more implants in posterior zone sites. The planned protocol change also recognized the simulated hammer-and-anvil adverse loading risk as a likely resultant disparity between uncontrollable occlusal forces and otherwise vulnerable recipient bone sites (Fig 9-17).

An alternative approach was to apply a version of the original protocol but compensate for any shortcomings in specific situations (Fig 9-18). For example, in anatomically unfavorable

**Fig 9-16** Expansion of the initial somewhat formulaic approach (a) gradually evolved into decisions to recruit more widespread implant distribution (b, d, and e) with added scope for optimal esthetic results (c and f), especially where a generous smile was present.

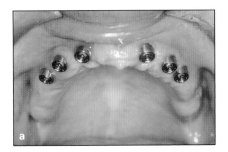
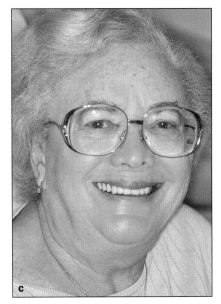
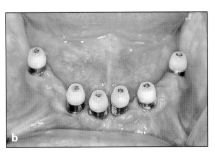
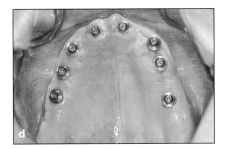
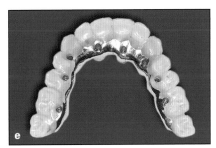
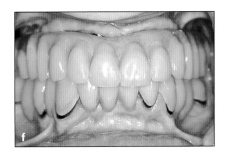

maxillary posterior zones and in the face of patient reluctance to undergo more sophisticated surgery, an anterior implant-supported fixed prosthesis could be combined with a removable posterior one (Fig 9-19). This approach remains a prudent one whenever bilateral pneumatization of the maxillary sinuses precludes a posterior surgical intervention and an anterior fixed prosthesis is demanded.

Overdenture designs were initially resorted to when an insufficient number of implants were available to support a fixed prosthesis. However, it quickly became apparent that, in such situations, the overdenture permitted a more expedient and readily controlled esthetic outcome, and it was adopted as an extremely efficacious and economically attractive way of converting maladaptive complete-denture experiences to adaptive ones (Figs 9-20 to 9-23).

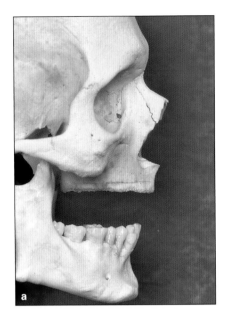 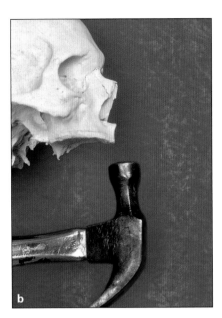

**Fig 9-17** *(a and b)* The hammer-and-anvil effect is a useful analogy for the clinician to keep in mind when treatment planning for the edentulous maxilla with implants.

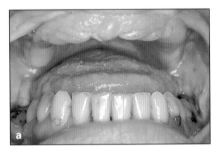 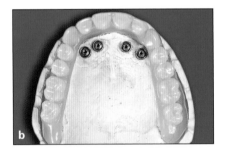

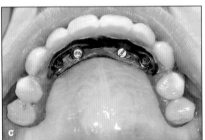 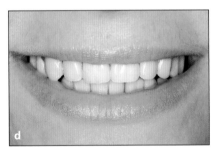

**Fig 9-18** Occasionally a dramatic departure from the traditional numeric formula is warranted (eg, when six or more teeth need to be replaced in the maxilla). *(a to d)* In this patient, a fixed prothesis with a shortened dental arch, as opposed to an overdenture design, was selected.

**Fig 9-19** *(a and b)* A somewhat similar challenge to that shown in Fig 9-18 was addressed by combining an anterior fixed prosthesis with a removable posterior one. This design was necessary because of the wide smile and the patient's refusal to undergo additional posterior site improvement surgery.

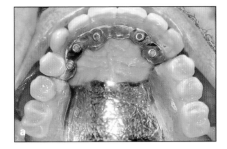 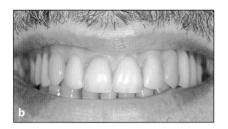

**Fig 9-20** *(a and b)* The versatility of the overdenture design is suggested in this clinical example and those in Figs 9-21 to 9-23.

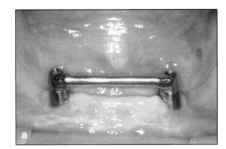 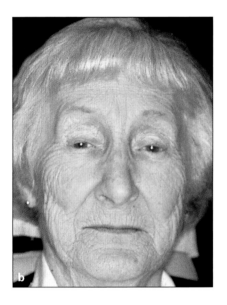

**Fig 9-21** *(near right)* Optimal control of esthetics achieved using the overdenture design.

**Fig 9-22** *(far right)* The overdenture design offers relative ease of technical fabrication because of the similarities to complete denture fabrication.

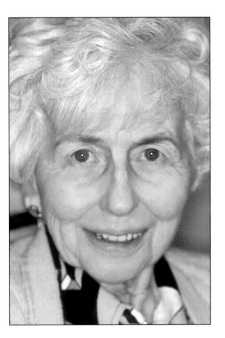 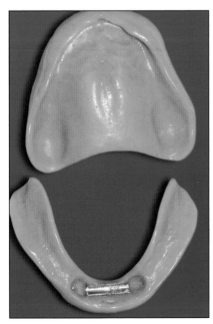

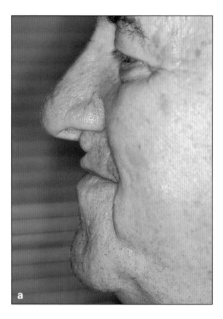

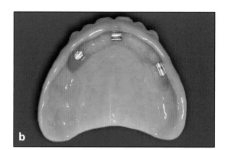

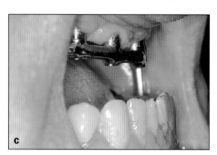

**Fig 9-23** *(a to c)* The overdenture is ideal for special morphologic situations such as an edentulous maxilla in a patient with a prognathic jaw relationship.

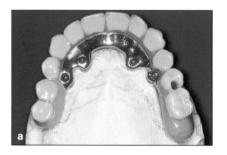

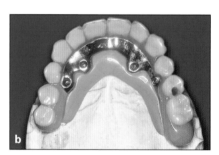

**Fig 9-24** Palatal space underneath a prosthesis *(a)* can cause speech problems, which are readily rectified with provisional or permanent wear of a customized obturator *(b)*.

## Speech problems

A few patients encounter speech articulation problems with their fixed implant-supported prostheses because the space under the prosthesis on the palatal side cannot be readily tolerated. It is prudent to inform all patients seeking maxillary treatment that transient speech articulation problems may be encountered. Rarely, complaints about minor but lingering alterations in speech articulation may persist, and an acrylic resin horseshoe-shaped palatal obturator may have to be provided (Fig 9-24); for an even fewer number of patients, the fixed prosthesis may have to be converted to an overdenture.

It could be argued that prescription of an overdenture design will preclude any problems with speech adaptation, irrespective of whether palatal coverage is included in the final prosthesis design. However, because there are no specific pretreatment indications for deciding who might not be able to adapt to a fixed design, and speech maladaptation is an infrequent outcome, the design choice is mainly based on the feasibility or desirability of the final number of abutments available for support in the context of patient choice.

## Flanges

The frequently encountered shrinkage of the edentulous maxilla's perimeter follows a predictable pattern. Sagittal and horizontal residual ridge reduction demand implant placement palatal to the final tooth positioning. Labial and buccal acrylic resin flanges are therefore needed to support lips and cheeks and to create the required overlying soft tissue seals for restored functional (eg, speech and bolus control) and esthetic integrity (Figs 9-25 and 9-26). Although necessary, such flange design will impose additional hygiene demands, and scrupulous care and massage of the peri-implant gingival tissues must be demonstrated to the patient and repeatedly reinforced.

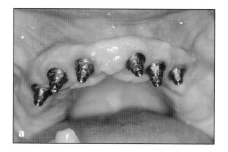
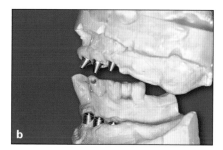
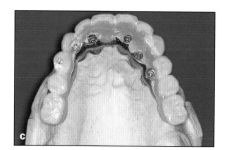

**Fig 9-25** *(a to f)* The use of a labial flange ensures optimal upper lip support and an overall esthetically pleasing result. This is often the only way to address the spatial disparity between implant placement in resorbed residual ridges and the required optimal prosthetic teeth placement.

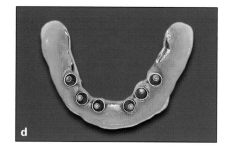
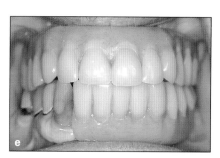
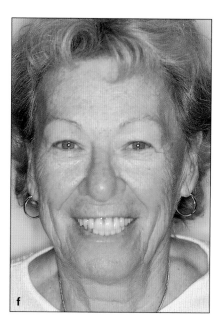

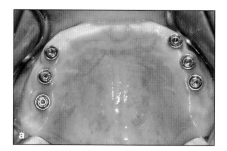
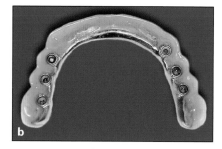
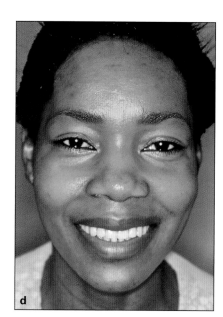

**Fig 9-26** *(a to d)* The labial flange augments optimal anterior tooth arrangement for function and esthetics.

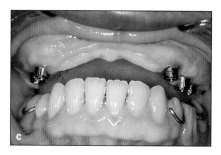

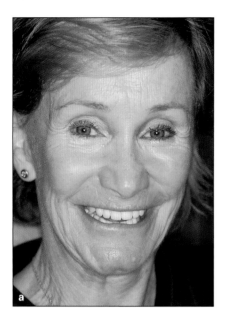

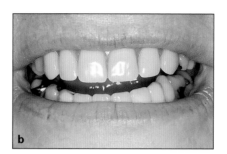

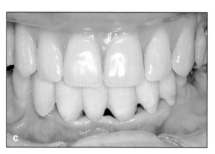

**Fig 9-27** Esthetic demands at the residual ridge level tend to be less challenging in the mandible than in the maxilla (see Figs 9-25 and 9-26) since mandibular labial activity *(a and b)* remains the final determinant of the hygiene-driven design for the access areas around each peri-implant site *(c)*.

An esthetically and functionally acceptable flange design is more critical in maxillary prostheses than in mandibular ones. It is determined by evaluation of upper lip activities, the patient's assessment regarding speech articulation as well as salivary leakage (sometimes described as "spraying" while talking), and the need to access the peri-implant gingival sites for home care hygiene. The reconciliation of all three objectives may not always be achieved immediately and may need fine-tuning over an initial trial period.

As a rule, the maxillary flange successfully addresses labial and cheek support needs while ensuring very respectable esthetics. However, this may not always be easy to prognosticate, and the overdenture protocol becomes a prudent alternative when esthetic support, adequate prosthesis retention, and ease of home care take priority over the demand for a fixed prosthodontic solution.

The mandibular fixed prosthesis offers relatively few design challenges, particularly because the space underneath the labial flange is rarely an esthetic problem. Experience suggests that even the most extreme lower lip movement rarely exposes the space between the labial flange on the prosthesis and the gingival tissues. The planned space is designed to facilitate oral hygiene protocols, and the resultant gingival "black triangle" or "black rectangle" will rarely cause a patient more than a minor inconvenience with food trapping and does not create an esthetic concern in the mandible (Figs 9-27 to 9-29). Similar spaces in the maxilla may have to be addressed if they cause a patient anxiety (Fig 9-30).

Food entrapment may be a concern with both maxillary and mandibular overdentures, more particularly if traditional objectives in complete-denture design and construction are not observed.

## Gingival esthetics

Time-dependent residual ridge resorption often takes its toll on residual ridge morphology, which in turn demands a reconciliation of implant placement with the location of the prosthetic tooth arrangement. An optimal esthetic result will then require the recruitment of traditional fixed and removable partial denture laboratory technology.

If the plan is to select porcelain teeth, the equivalent of a complete-arch metal-ceramic prostheses is fabricated. Alternatively, a titanium frame can also be produced through computer-aided design and machining. In this case, individual porcelain crowns are for individual cementation on the posts that are designed on the frame. This design tends to be restricted to situations where minimal residual ridge reduction has occurred, and the objective is to have the replacement teeth look as if they are emerging from the gingival tissues. This goal makes for a somewhat demanding surgical responsibility, because the prosthesis design must mask the location of the implants without sacrificing ideal tooth positioning.

When the residual ridge morphology has been quantitatively compromised, the framework is also recruited into

**Fig 9-28** *(a to c)* Images underscore the importance of reconciling circumoral activity with the desired esthetic result and ongoing hygiene access considerations. Whenever plaque accumulation and staining were evident, the prosthesis was removed, ultrasonically cleaned, and laboratory polished. In this patient and the one shown in Fig 9-29, clinical follow-ups of more than two decades ensured an optimal soft tissue picture, although it was apparent that implant placement in this patient was crowded.

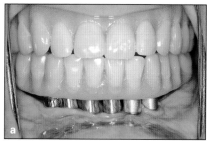
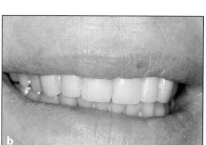
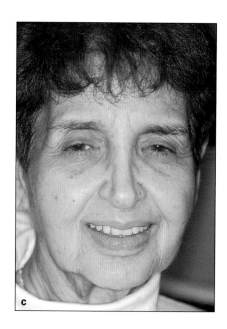

**Fig 9-29** *(a and b)* Another patient in which circumoral activity was balanced with esthetics and the need for hygiene access.

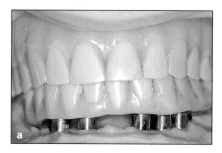
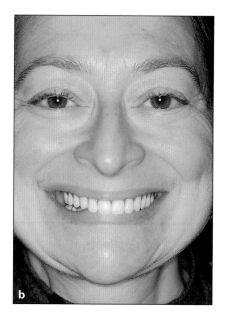

**Fig 9-30** *(a)* The occasional occurrence of a so-called black triangle in an anterior site may be a cause of concern. *(b)* Such occurrences are not always readily managed with an acrylic resin flange if an unfavorable smile line is present. However, better prosthetic design treatment planning (eg, alterations in adjacent teeth morphologies) can frequently avoid this unfortunate sort of contingency.

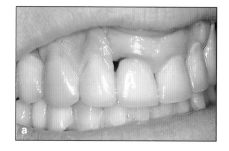
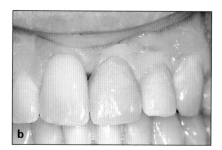

carrying a gingival analog. This technique is borrowed from the removable partial denture laboratory design format and is a versatile and relatively inexpensive method. It also lends itself to an even more customized esthetic design if the computer-designed framework is planned to accommodate incorporation of both gingival analogs and individual crown replacements. It is a far more expensive approach, albeit not necessarily a superior one. Like many prosthodontic treatment design options, this method reflects the range of high-technology sophistication that continues to play a major role in prosthodontic decision making.

## Ethical considerations

The merits of implant-supported overdentures catalyzed the popular conviction that the technique should be regarded as the standard of care for managing edentulism, particularly mandibular edentulism. This consideration is discussed in chapter 12 but demands some clinical management observations here.

There seems to be little doubt that concerns with stability and retention confront the vast majority of denture-wearers, particularly over time. These concerns are reported as readily rectified if an overdenture is prescribed, and it has become very tempting to seek to place a couple of implants under each mandibular denture. It could also be argued that, in the long term, residual ridge resorption would be reduced and esthetic requirements would be more readily addressed, especially if moderate to advanced bone changes have already occurred. There are financial implications as well. Therefore, each treatment decision must be influenced by a reconciliation of the many factors that impact individual patient-mediated needs and the health professional's concerns.

## Conclusions

The profession remains unsure about optimal treatment design specifics, notably the number of implants and the methods of securing mechanical stability and retention. Numerous variations on these themes have been proposed. Although they all seem rational and clinically acceptable, a number of tentative conclusions can also be reached from a synthesis of the available literature on the subjects:

- Two or at most three implants provide very satisfactory results for the vast majority of successfully managed mandibular overdentures. If more secure retention is desired, the number of implants can always be increased. The latter circumstance would then make the implant support almost identical to the support offered by the design of a fixed prosthesis.
- A minimum of three or four implants is recommended for the maxilla; the inclusion of extra implant support is dictated by occlusal considerations and the choice to recruit the hard palate for additional prosthetic support.
- Implant distribution in either arch should be as widespread and in some cases as symmetric as possible.
- The mechanical methods of providing retention are both versatile and numerous; they cover a range of ingenious designs, from studs to bars to magnets. When used correctly they invariably offer gratifying results for the vast majority of patients. Occasionally an initially prescribed method will not satisfy a patient's expectations, and the retentive components may have to be augmented or even changed. Debate as to the best attachment mechanism appears to be an extension of the debate that has raged on over the years in the area of removable partial dentures vis-à-vis clasp and precision attachment designs.
- The choice of a bar and clip assembly lends itself to a wide range of bar designs, including straight, curved, cantilevered, or separate segments. The diversity of possible forms reflects design ingenuity coupled with retentive and space requirements and hygiene considerations (Fig 9-31).
- For some patients, their efforts at home care and the wear and tear to which they subject their prostheses may necessitate frequent and meticulous maintenance service. The situation is not unlike what most clinicians encounter routinely with a segment of patients in routine prosthodontic practices. Even with implant prosthodontic treatment, and its implied ecologic advantages, the relationship between patient behaviors and the nature of the clinical intervention must be carefully monitored.

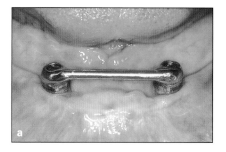
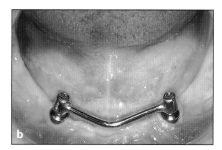
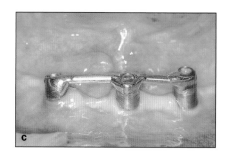
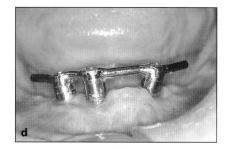
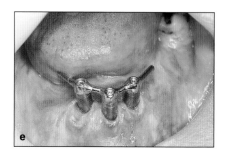
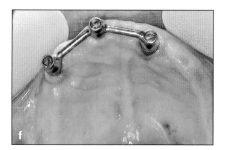
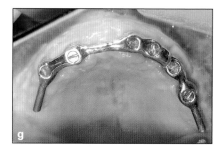

**Fig 9-31** Examples of different mandibular *(a to e)* and maxillary *(f and g)* bar design. These are a few of the numerous ingenious variations developed for prosthetic retention in overdentures. The variations result from diverse morphologic dictates encountered together with technical space considerations and ultimately the dentist's and technician's judgment calls.

# Protocols for Partially Edentulous Patients

## Missing multiple teeth in anterior zones

Management of Class IV partial edentulism with implants was a logical and lateral treatment move from the edentulous experience that emphasized the anterior and esthetic zones of both arches. These sites are frequently favorable ones on both quantitative and qualitative grounds because the presence of adjacent teeth has probably contributed to the relative preservation of the width and height of residual bone in the anterior zone. Yet the sites are also accompanied by fewer examples of anatomic challenges, which are more frequently encountered in posterior zones (Fig 9-32). It is also not surprising, therefore, that the implant technique has rapidly eclipsed the use of the classic six- to eight-unit fixed partial denture whenever multiple anterior teeth are missing, particularly if residual ridge resorption has been minimal or traumatic tooth avulsion has oc-

curred with very limited residual ridge damage. The implant protocol also has become a very viable alternative to a removable partial denture (Figs 9-33 to 9-38).

This section highlights a number of critical points in the management of Class IV partial edentulism, particularly in the maxilla.

## Occlusal forces

Available bilateral natural or restored posterior occlusal support usually offers favorable scope for optimal planning to avoid potentially adverse occlusal loading. A neutral incisal guidance can be incorporated to reduce load distribution on implant support in the horizontal plane. This ensures a reduction in the risk of higher bending moments on the implants and the consequent increase in the interfacial stress concentration. This ability to control the distribution of adverse occlusal forces by largely restricting them to posterior natural or restored dentitions may very well be an additional reason for the high success rates reported in this zone.

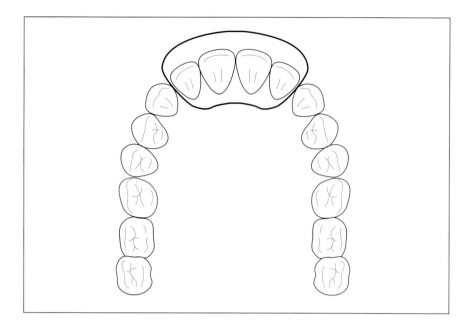

**Fig 9-32** Kennedy Class IV partial edentulism may present unique anatomic and associated esthetic challenges for restoration, depending upon the final shape of the edentulous site. This in turn impacts incisal guidance considerations in the initial treatment planning stages with trial teeth setups.

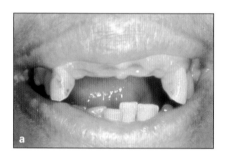
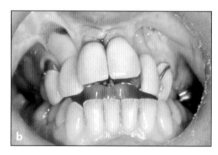
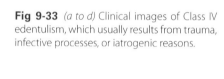

**Fig 9-33** *(a to d)* Clinical images of Class IV edentulism, which usually results from trauma, infective processes, or iatrogenic reasons.

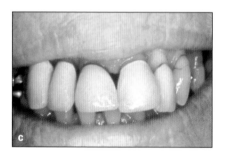
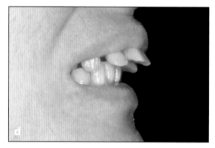

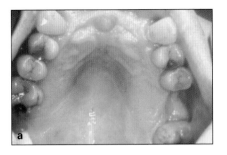
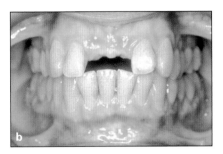
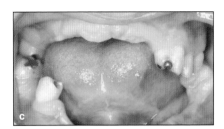
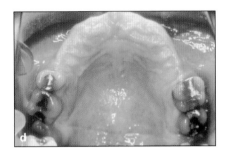
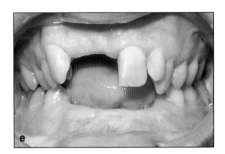

**Fig 9-34** *(a to e)* The resultant size of the residual edentulous tissues in Class IV sites varies in three dimensions.

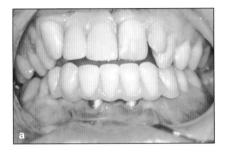
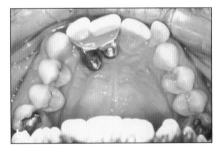
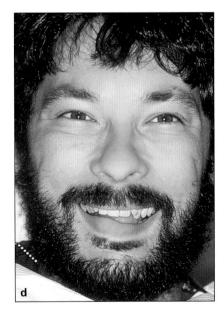
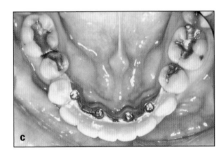

**Fig 9-35** *(a to d)* Class IV edentulism can be readily restored without significant surgical intervention.

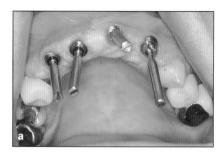

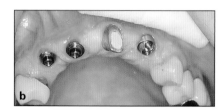

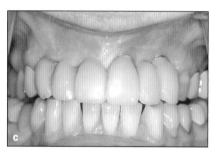

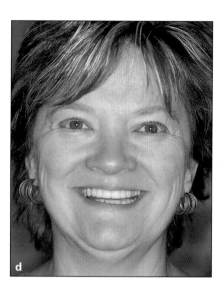

**Fig 9-36** *(a to d)* Careful surgical planning and choice of abutment ensures predictably good results.

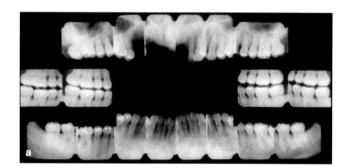

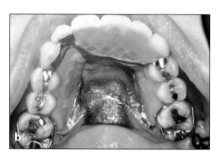

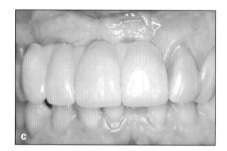

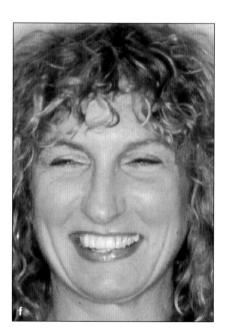

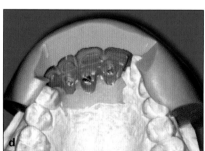

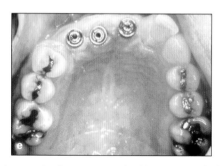

**Fig 9-37** Case history wherein anterior teeth and supporting bone were avulsed in a motor vehicle accident *(a)*. The original removable partial denture *(b and c)* served as an esthetic template *(d)* for the provision of an implant-supported fixed partial denture with interproximal porcelain of simulated gingival tissue *(e and f)* to provide a continuum of esthetic satisfaction for the patient.

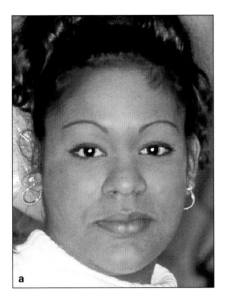

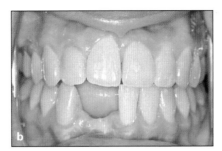

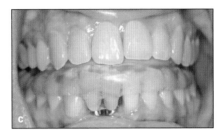

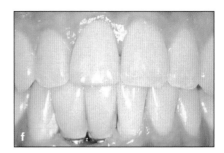

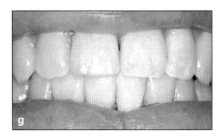

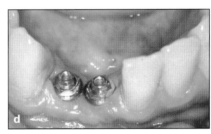

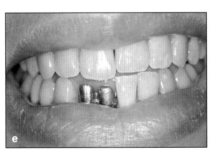

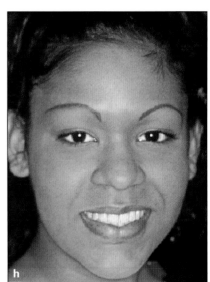

**Fig 9-38** *(a to e)* Example of using a surgical template with two prosthetic teeth to guide the placement of the required anterior mandibular implants. *(f to h)* The surgical positioning ensured crown placement that provided the desired result in an overall context of circumoral activities.

This experience permits the prescription of up to four prosthetic pontics supported by just two or more implants, as determined by space availability. This in turn has a bearing on the planning of the final esthetic outcome, particularly when the planned prosthetic teeth are meant to simulate emergence from a virtually unresorbed residual ridge.

## Esthetics

The major challenge in treating Class IV partial edentulism is esthetics. It demands a reconciliation of morphologic and functional dictates with esthetic objectives and design hard-

ware. The patient's smile line is the key determinant, with a revealing smile line demanding the following considerations:

• If a labial flange is not required and a natural tooth emergence profile is mandatory, the number and placement of implants and location of prosthetic teeth must be impeccably controlled. The challenge is similar to that in routine anterior fixed partial denture designs; in this case, it is rendered somewhat more demanding by the need for absolutely accurate implant surgical location. Consequently, a patient-approved trial tooth setup must precede accurate surgical

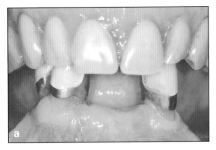
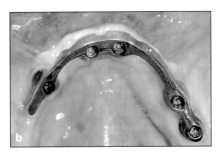
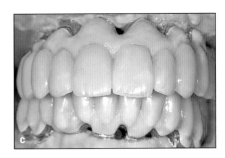

**Fig 9-39** With consummate skill, certain dental technicians can create exceptional analogs for missing gingival tissues. The maxillary complete denture *(a)* and mandibular removable partial denture have been replaced via a customized bar in the maxilla *(b)* and a combination of implant- and tooth-supported prostheses *(c)*. (Courtesy of Dr Kenneth Malament.)

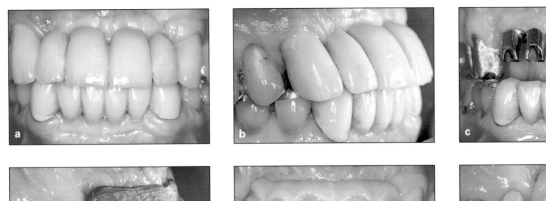
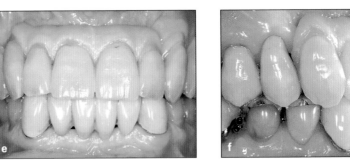
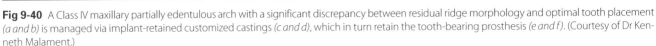

**Fig 9-40** A Class IV maxillary partially edentulous arch with a significant discrepancy between residual ridge morphology and optimal tooth placement *(a and b)* is managed via implant-retained customized castings *(c and d)*, which in turn retain the tooth-bearing prosthesis *(e and f)*. (Courtesy of Dr Kenneth Malament.)

splint production, which must then be conscientiously employed during the surgical procedure. Component design (customized or angulated abutments) also permits compensation for small surgical discrepancies that result in tilted implants. The indispensable partnership of experienced dental technicians is unquestionable in situations that fall outside the routine planned surgical/prosthodontic synergies.

- If a labial flange is required (where moderate to advanced residual ridge resorption has occurred) implant placement is palatal to the prosthetic teeth, and the challenge is to have the labial gingival analog match adjacent natural tissues, which is not an easy or routine task. This challenge is often solved with the use of ceramic, as opposed to acrylic resin, flanges (Figs 9-39 and 9-40).

**Fig 9-41** Kennedy classification of partial edentulism. The management of posterior zone partial edentulism with implants evolved from the proven efficacy and effectiveness experiences in the anterior zones, notably with the edentulous experience.

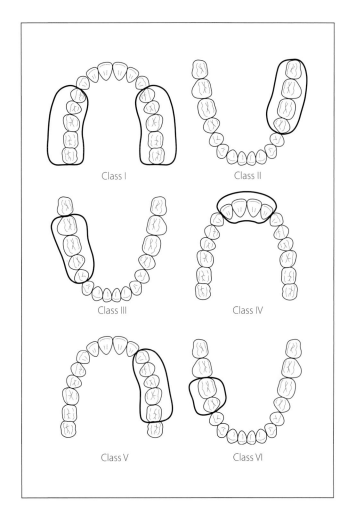

Class I

Class II

Class III

Class IV

Class V

Class VI

## Missing multiple teeth in posterior zones

Multiple tooth loss in the posterior zones (Fig 9-41), particularly if a distal abutment is not present, used to be routinely managed with removable partial dentures or in special situations with unilateral or bilateral cantilevered pontics attached to splinted crowns placed on the anterior residual dentition.

Alternatively, the concept of a shortened dental arch was applied, in spite of its inherent esthetic and possibly even functional time-dependent shortcomings. In recent years, a strong scientific endorsement of the success of implant-supported tooth replacements in the posterior zones has permitted inclusion of the implant technique for this frequently challenging clinical predicament (Figs 9-42 and 9-43).

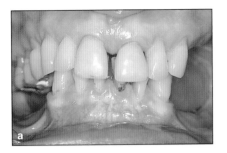
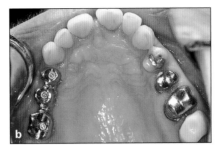
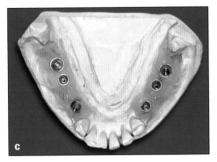
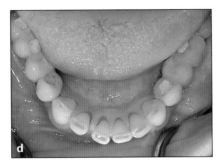
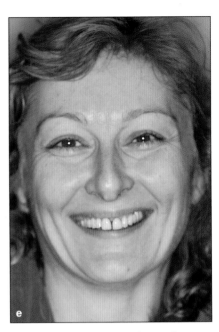

**Fig 9-42** Improved imaging of posterior zones and their unique anatomic landmarks, combined with technologic improvements and surgical ingenuity, have enabled surgeons to exploit the maxillary sinuses for additional implant placement via sinus lift protocols. *(a)* Pretreatment. *(b)* A reflected occlusal view of the maxillary arch following implant placement on the left side and placement of copings on the right molars, which have been significantly reduced after endodontic treatment. Occlusal views of the master cast *(c)* and the prostheses in place *(d)* are supplemented with a recall photograph *(e)*.

## Imaging

The profession's ability to reliably image and more thoroughly assess proposed host sites has grown exponentially as a result of significant advances in radiographic imaging (Fig 9-44; also see chapter 6). Three-dimensional images of bone quantity and quality are now indispensable surgical planning tools and reveal both the height and width of selected sites. Both measurements ensure accurate location of the inferior alveolar canal contents and reveal the possible significance of the ratio of implant volume to remaining bone volume. These measurements help to determine the length and width of a suitable implant for the site (Fig 9-45). Moreover, this choice could be a predictor of a successful long-term outcome.

## Implant selection

The original formula, five or six 10-mm-long implants in anterior zones to support complete-arch replacements, had to be substantially modified to address the restricted dimensions of posterior edentulous spans. The restrictions were both vertical and horizontal, but the implant industry very rapidly produced diverse sizes to accommodate most residual host bone dimensions. Moreover, ongoing surgical ingenuity introduced block onlay grafting techniques, sinus lifts, ridge splitting, lateralization of nerve canal contents, and distraction osteogenesis to provide a better host site match for the different implant sizes.

Such innovations helped to expand the indications for implant treatment in these zones, even if the proposed and exciting repertoire of preprosthetic surgical interventions is not yet supported by long-term outcome studies. It appears that three implants are better than two in these zones and that longer implants are preferable to shorter ones. It has also been reported that one or two implants can be attached to natural healthy abutment teeth (preferably canines) to avoid the need for additional implants or to avoid additional surgical site preparation. Consequently, mix of implant sizes and numbers, based on individual anatomic dictates, becomes the prudent modus operandi. Furthermore, offsetting the implant locations whenever ridge width permits is encouraged; earlier concerns regarding tilted implants or nonaxial loading situations have been largely negated by extensive clinical experience.

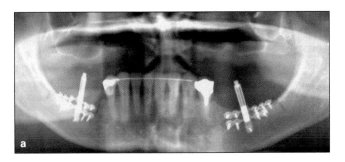

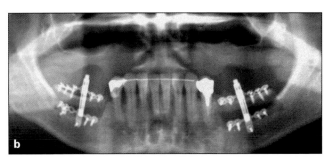

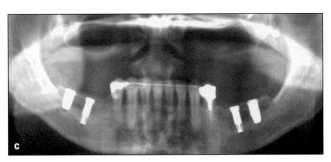

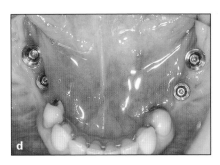

**Fig 9-43** Another surgical innovation for management of posterior partial edentulism, particularly in the mandible, is the distraction osteogenesis technique for vertical bone height augmentation. This procedure was carried out successfully several years ago in this middle-aged patient. *(a to c)* The panoramic radiographs illustrate the bony distraction sequence leading up to the bilaterally placed osseointegrated implants. *(d and e)* Clinical prosthodontic sequence. *(f and g)* Treatment completion. (Courtesy of Dr David Walker, Univeristy of Toronto.)

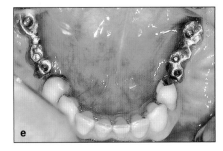

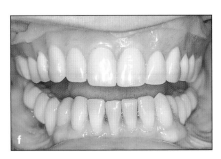

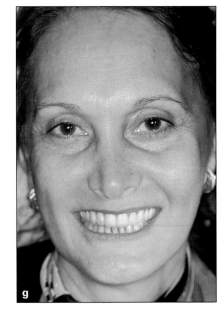

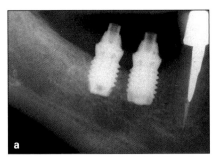

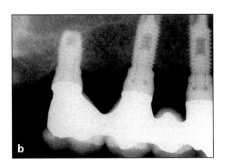

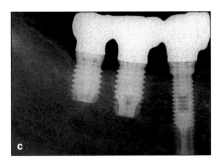

**Fig 9-44** *(a to c)* Significant advances in imaging techniques (as described in chapter 6) have improved the ability to assess three-dimensional bone quantity and quality beyond the early two-dimensional periapical images.

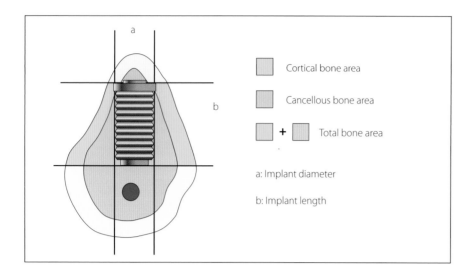

**Fig 9-45** Research suggests that successful treatment outcomes with wide-bodied implants may be related to aspects of the ratio between host bone and actual implant dimensions. This ratio may impact the quality of the induced osseointegration. The cumulative success rate of 5.0-mm-diameter wide-platform implants was reported to be lower than that of regular-diameter implants, which seems to be related to a higher ratio of implant–host bone dimensions, suggesting that the dimension of the host bone site may influence an implant's osseointegrated outcome. Further multivariate analyses should be undertaken to confirm this hypothesis. (Courtesy of Professor Snag-Wan Shin.)

Roughened implant surfaces suggest earlier and perhaps even better interfacial healing responses. This would in turn permit a one-stage surgery and perhaps even early- or immediate-loading protocols. However, the latter approach does need more compelling documentation before it can be regarded as a recommended routine protocol.

## Potential failure

Much doubt has been expressed (certainly in this book) about the presumption that patients with a history of periodontal disease may not be good candidates for osseointegration. Because posterior tooth loss is frequently the result of periodontal disease, it might seem logical to avoid implant treatment if a patient's history of tooth loss involved periodontal disease. However, the pathogenesis of this infective process and the suspected causes of implant failure do not appear to be identical. The combination of compromised healing and adverse loading appears to be the major concern, and all treatment planning must reconcile and address the several aspects of the associated biologic challenge of the osseointegration process if a successful outcome is to be achieved. For further discussion of osseointegration failure, see chapter 11.

## *Missing single tooth*

Excellent results with osseointegration in replacing complete or partial dentitions led to a rapid extrapolation of published results and inferred success for single-tooth implants. This oc-

curred in spite of lingering concerns about important issues that continue to influence the current protocols. The concerns are still relevant, although it is popularly believed that clinical experience has now solved most of them.

## Mechanical considerations

A reliable quantification of the "holding power" (or efficacy of osseointegration) of the individual implant in diverse sites of either jaw is not available. The quantifiable optimal ratio of cancellous host bone volume to implant size that would ensure the desired support for even the most adverse occlusal loading on the single coronal replacement remains elusive. It is clear that long-term favorable outcomes for multiple splinted implants cannot be automatically extrapolated to single implants; in other words, the loading limits of the single implant are unknown. Dentists have addressed this concern through prudent occlusal design planning for the single crown in the context of anticipated differences in future loading magnitudes, durations, and frequencies. A desire to protect the single implant as much as possible by minimizing or even precluding occlusal crown contacts, particularly in excursive positions, has been intuitively applied.

In fact, it has been tempting to categorize the single implant as being a reliable and esthetically elegant space maintainer that also happens to be a very ecologically sound replacement for a missing tooth. Furthermore, the screw-retained crown is retrievable and repairable, should it be chipped; it can also be readily modified over the years to alter its appearance and dimensions.

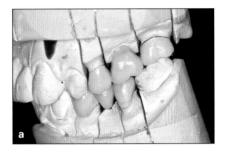

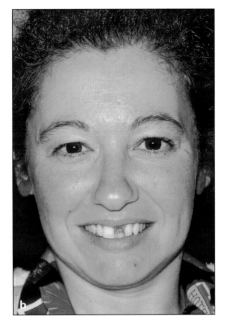

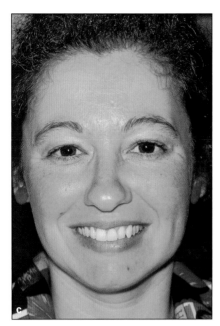

**Fig 9-46** The entry-level technical and clinical efforts associated with a traditional, ecologically compromising three-unit fixed prosthesis *(a)* have been largely eclipsed by the single-implant–supported crown *(b and c)*.

The technique's introduction has rung a virtual death knell for the traditional three-unit fixed partial denture, which until recently was the backbone of undergraduate prosthodontic programs in most dental schools (Fig 9-46). In spite of this important ecologic treatment advance, it must be emphasized that no comparison is available between full loading, partial loading, and nonloading for single implants in different jaw sites in patients with different parafunctional behavioral histories. The result is the inevitable if misleading rationalizations of occlusal planning when dealing with anterior and posterior locations for single implants.

Clinical experience suggests the following: A single implant's dimensions should not "crowd" the available host cancellous bone site, nor should it be overwhelmed by the available bone volume. The current availability of mechanically reliable narrow and wide implants from several manufacturers permits optimal reconciliation of site volume, implant dimensions, and anticipated loading scenarios for most clinical situations.

## Bone loss

Several publications have reported annual marginal bone loss around single implants to be less than 0.2 mm per year after the first year of loading. These values are comparable to published results from other long-term outcome studies in edentulous and partially edentulous patients and augur well for the technique. However, changes appear to be more likely in alveolar bone than in basal bone. Consequently it must be remembered that in younger patients, and particularly in conspicuously visible sites, resultant gingival recessions will occur and may indeed lead to esthetic challenges in the long term. Prosthodontic revisions will be necessary, and young patients in particular should be prepared for such maintenance care. Esthetics is unlikely to be a problem in association with bone loss around posterior replacements because the location frequently precludes eventual cervical visibility of the restoration.

Furthermore, popularly employed plastic surgical procedures and site development techniques are still unaccompanied by rigorously documented long-term outcome information regarding their impact on stable cervical bone levels around single implants. Consequently, the current repertoire of surgical innovations, commercially proposed regenerative techniques, and different abutment materials and designs must be regarded with caution (perhaps even skepticism) because they may turn out to be long on claims of efficacy but short on time-dependent veracity.

## Esthetics

Numerous studies have endorsed patient satisfaction with implant-supported single crowns, although it is clear that patients and dentists have different criteria for evaluating dental care as well as esthetic results. For example, studies have reported that no single factor used in multiple regression analysis influenced patients' satisfaction with the appearance of a crown to a statistically significant level, and that an individual patient's concept of esthetic appearance differs substantially from that of a dentist. Factors considered to be significant by professionals may not be regarded as being of decisive importance by patients.

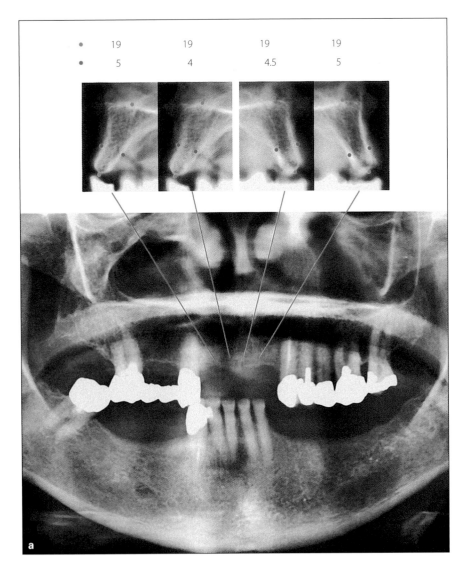

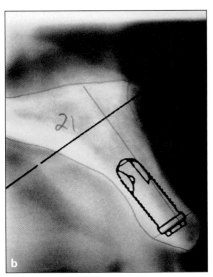

**Fig 9-47** Tomographic views of anterior maxillary sites reveal both sagittal congruency *(a)* and incongruency *(b)* between dimensions of the host site and implants. *(a)* Length *(green dots)* and width *(red dots)* measurements are made to determine optimal implant dimensions for the potential host sites. *(b)* The implant selected is clearly not a good choice. The considerable variance in bone histology that exists even in the same field and the same section reflects the functional plasticity of alveolar bone as it adapts to the many forms of stress imposed on it.

Nonetheless, these considerations do not necessarily take full cognizance of the subtle relationship between the prosthetic crown and its surrounding soft tissues, because the overall esthetic evaluation involves more than exclusive focus on the crown replacement. As a result, dentist-mediated concerns about gingival appearance in terms of both its dimensions and contours have expanded clinical understanding of this much localized yet highly relevant concern. Chapter 8 offers a synthesis of current information on some unique soft tissue considerations, but key points that deserve highlighting are also discussed in this chapter.

The suitability of a proposed host bone site for single implant placement is determined by its health status and the quantity and quality of the available host bed. Less-than-ideal quality alone is not necessarily an insurmountable challenge, thanks to readily acquired surgical skills as well as good judg-

ment in site preparation and loading protocols. The surgical decision is also influenced by the site's three-dimensional morphology, because esthetic considerations (particularly in the exposed anterior zones) might necessitate a so-called site enhancement intervention to improve the esthetic integrity of the circumimplant soft tissue. Therefore, a surgeon is frequently confronted with the decision regarding whether an implant can be placed in the native bone site with or without the need for an enhancement procedure.

As a rule, residual ridge dimensions result from a time-dependent bone reduction process related to the etiology of the tooth loss. The resultant potential implant site is also influenced by the predictable direction of the resorptive process in accordance with the original orientation of the tooth roots and their periodontal ligaments. Consequently in the anterior zone the sagittal and horizontal profiles of sockets heal in an

---

**Box 9-3** SURGICAL LOCATION OF THE SINGLE IMPLANT AND ATTENDANT CONSIDERATIONS FOLLOWING TOOTH LOSS

1. The implant is placed directly in the tooth socket along the same long axis as the tooth (see Fig 9-48). This decision may be accompanied by:
   - *Incompatibility between the socket and implant size, which may compromise implant stability*
   - *Resultant gaps that may have to be filled with native bone particles or substitute*
   - *The need for angulated or customized abutments*

2. The implant is placed as vertically as possible with adequate bone surrounding it. Two clinical examples (see Figs 9-49 and 9-50) illustrate resultant slight gingival cervical convexity above/below the crown. This is managed by:
   - *Gingival stretching or plumping*
   - *Soft tissue graft*
   - *No additional intervention, but reliance on clinical judgment and explanation to patient*

3. The implant is placed palatally/lingually and therefore distant from the actual esthetic location of the crown adjacent to the natural teeth (see Fig 9-51). This approach is frequently precluded via site improvement through bone and/or soft tissue augmentation, especially if the bony indentation is sufficiently severe. It can, however, also be addressed by:
   - *A ridge-lapped pontic if a waxup try-in endorses the esthetic outcome. This is arguably an underappreciated alternative, although it demands scrupulous home care to avoid an unfavorably altered gingival picture. Furthermore, the overlying bony indentation must be only a mild one.*
   - *Pontic camouflage or use of a gingival analog (least desirable option since it is not easily or predictably achieved).*

---

upward and palatal direction in the maxilla and in a downward and lingual direction in the mandible. The same occurs in the posterior maxillary zone, but not in the posterior mandibular zone. In the posterior mandible, the reduction is in a buccal horizontal direction.

The general predictability regarding the direction of residual ridge reduction was initially studied in edentulous patients, with the early and impressive research of Tallgren, Atwood, and Carlsson laying down the groundwork for an understanding of bone morphologic outcomes. The current availability of tomographic imaging has added a new dimension to the study of small or even individual edentulous sites. As a result, considerable attention has focused on the surgical planning and esthetic outcome concerns related to individual tooth replacement with an implant-supported crown. Figure 9-47 illustrates this challenge in the sense that the sagittal dimensions of the

proposed host bone sites may not routinely permit accommodation of an implant's circumferential dimension. Recalling the histologic features of these sites provides a better understanding of the rationale for clinical interventions. The alveolar process consists of alveolar bone, which is partially or completely lost when a tooth is extracted. This alveolar bone contains the sockets, which are lined by bundle bone (often called a *lamina dura* by radiologists), the bulk of which is extremely variable. Consequently sagittal views of proposed individual implant sites demonstrate a spectrum of morphologic variations that can challenge the surgical ingenuity required for site improvement or else preclude its use entirely.

There are three general possibilities for anterior maxillary resorptive patterns (Box 9-3), and each is addressed with popular compensatory surgical technique initiatives (Figs 9-48 to 9-51). The initiatives need not, and should not, be routine

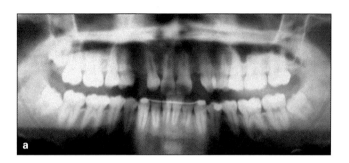

**Fig 9-48** *(a to c)* Panoramic radiographs pre- and postorthodontic implant treatment of congenitally missing teeth. *(d and e)* The three-dimensional morphology of the selected implant sites demanded implant placement in a long axis that simulated their placement in fresh extraction sockets. The resultant long axes for the simulated roots required the use of one angulated and one customized abutment to achieve the desired esthetic result *(f to j)*.

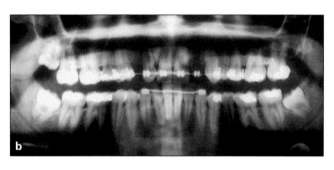

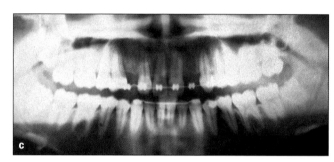

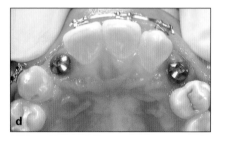

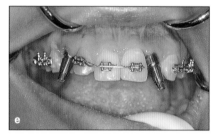

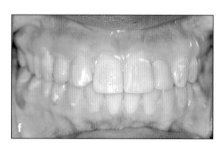

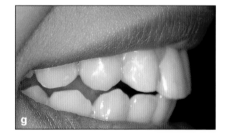

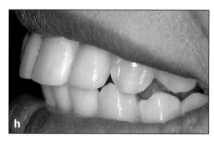

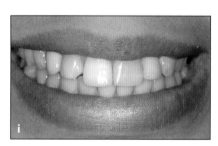

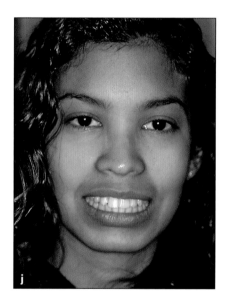

**Fig 9-49** *(a and b)* In a mandibular edentulous site resulting from an avulsed tooth, the implant is placed as vertically as possible with adequate bone surrounding it. This results in a slight offset necessitating a minor ridge lap between the crown's required position and the implant's actual long axis.

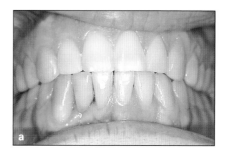

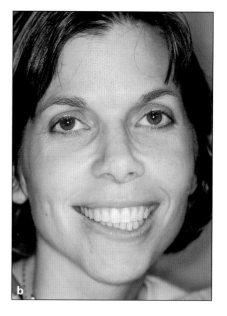

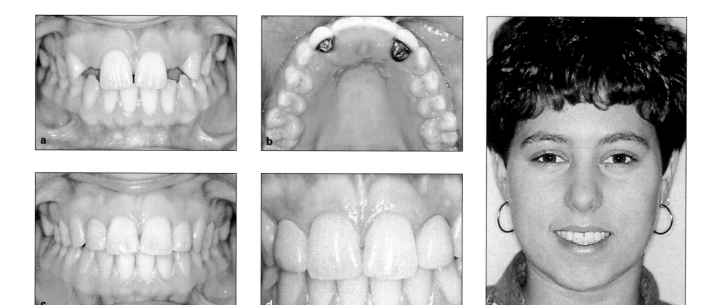

**Fig 9-50** Congenitally missing maxillary lateral incisors *(a)* are replaced with implants placed as vertically as possible *(b to e)* with labiogingival plumping, which ensures a better esthetic result.

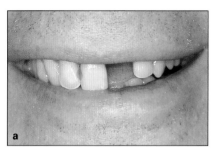 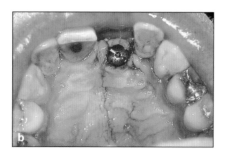 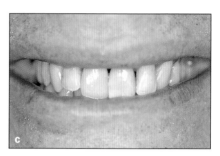

**Fig 9-51** *(a)* The left maxillary central incisor was lost because of advanced localized periodontal and endodontic disease. *(b)* The proposed host bone site was not improved or augmented at the patient's specific request, and the implant was placed palatally. *(c)* The prosthetic replacement ridge-lapped the residual ridge area to create the illusion of a normal emergence profile. Routine and simple home care protocols were assigned and regularly reinforced to ensure the maintenance of a stable and healthy soft tissue outcome.

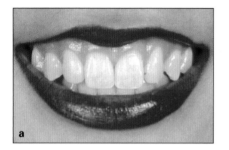

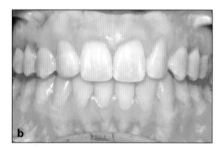

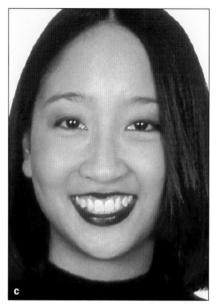

**Fig 9-52** *(a to c)* The brilliance of orthodontic management of congenitally missing laterals is displayed in this patient, who was a classically suitable candidate. The entire posterior dentition was moved forward bilaterally since minor morphologic alteration of the canines permitted their esthetic modification to occupy the new position of lateral incisors.

ones, because the major esthetic determinant remains an evaluation of labial morphology and extreme functional movement. Therefore, the current near epidemic of site improvement interventions need not be encouraged as an absolute pre–implant treatment necessity, just because the techniques are available and ingenious. In many cases, orthodontic management of the single anterior space can also yield impressive treatment results. Figure 9-52 is such an example, reconciling numerous pretreatment considerations—patient age and desire, morphologic features, occlusal considerations, and so on. In the end, patient-mediated concerns, guided by prudent professional clinical and ethical judgment, must never be usurped by fortuitous and even formulaic treatment agendas.

# RECOMMENDED READING

Attard NJ, Zarb GA. Long-term treatment outcomes in edentulous patients with implant-fixed prostheses: The Toronto study. Int J Prosthodont 2004;17:417–424.

Attard NJ, Zarb GA. Long-term treatment outcomes in edentulous patients with overdentures. Int J Prosthodont 2004;17:425-433.

Beyron H. Occlusion: Point of significance in planning restorative procedures. J Prosthet Dent 1973;30:641–652.

Beyron H. Optimal occlusion. Dent Clin North Am 1969;13:537–554.

Eckert SE, Meraw SJ, Cal E, Ow RK. Analysis of incidence and associated factors with fractured implants: A retrospective study. Int J Oral Maxillofac Implants 2000;15:662–667.

Eckert SE, Wollan PC. Retrospective review of 1170 endosseous implants placed in partially edentulous jaws. J Prosthet Dent 1998;79:415–421.

Hobkirk JA, Watson RM, Searson LJ. Introducing Dental Implants. New York: Churchill Livingstone, 2003.

Jemt T, Ahlberg G, Henriksson K, Bondevik O. Changes of anterior clinical crown height in patients provided with single-implant restorations after more than 15 years of follow-up. Int J Prosthodont 2006;19:455–461.

Lindh T. The Tooth-Implant Supported Prosthesis [thesis]. Sweden: Umea University, 2001.

Naert I, Quirynen M. Surgical periodontal interventions: Long-term outcomes. Int J Prosthodont 2007;20:345–348.

Palacci P (ed). Esthetic Implant Dentistry: Soft and Hard Tissue Management. Chicago: Quintessence, 2001.

Rangert BPH, Krogh PH, Langer B, Van Roekel N. Bending overload and implant fracture: A retrospective clinical analysis. Int J Oral Maxillofac Implants 1995;10:326–334 [erratum 1996;11:575].

Renouard F, Rangert B. Risk Factors in Implant Dentistry: Simplified Clinical Analysis for Predictable Treatment, ed 2. Chicago: Quintessence, 2008.

Watzek G. Implants in Qualitatively Compromised Bone. Chicago: Quintessence, 2004.

Wennstrom JL, Ekestubbe A, Gröhndahl K, Karlsson S, Lindhe J. Oral rehabilitation with fixed partial dentures in periodontitis-susceptible subjects. A 5-year prospective study. J Clin Periodontol 2004;31:713–724.

Wyatt CL, Zarb GA. Treatment outcomes with implant-supported fixed partial dentures. Int J Oral Maxillofac Implants 1998;13:204–211.

Zarb GA, Bolender CL. Prosthodontic Treatment for Edentulous Patients: Complete Dentures and Implant-Supported Prostheses, ed 12. St Louis: Mosby, 2003.

Zarb JP, Zarb GA. Implant prosthodontic management of anterior partial edentulism: Long-term follow-up of a prospective study. J Can Dent Assoc 2002;68(2):92–96.

# EARLY-LOADING PROTOCOLS

Nikolai Attard | George A. Zarb

Previous chapters have identified surgical and prosthodontic determinants for long-term clinical success when the original two-stage osseointegration technique is used. This traditional protocol included a prudent, if somewhat arbitrarily determined, interval for the unloaded healing phase between the two surgical stages. In recent years, the fiscal and psychosocial implications of accelerated and presumably simpler osseointegration protocols catalyzed a demand for a modified clinical management timetable. The timing and sequence of the original protocol were reevaluated, alternative scenarios were proposed, and concepts of immediate- and early-loading protocols were introduced and popularized.

The key initiatives for this change resulted from a desire for quicker clinical solutions, combined with the promise of immediate implant stabilization suggested by new macroscopic and microscopic surface design features. A subtle but profound shift in the presumed outcome determinants of successful osseointegration occurred as the commercial promise of manufactured buzz phrases entered the dentist's success lexicon. Old protocols were quickly modified or even eclipsed because of the new claims for improved and more rapidly induced osseointegration. Some examples of commercial claims are self-evident in their clinical appeal:

- Active and hydrophilic surface technology
- Increased and early bone-to-implant contact
- Reduction in healing time
- Stimulation of bone growth as well as provision of bone preservation

While conceptually exciting and indeed frequently prescribed, the protocol change must be regarded as still at the trial stage, because its status for routine application is largely based on case history series reports, site-specific success outcomes, and perhaps most critically in relatively short-term studies.

Crucial questions should be answered before the protocol changes are universally adopted. Box 10-1 lists some of these concerns.

A frequently cited reason for the success of early-loading protocols is the implant's primary mechanical stability provided by microscopic or macroscopic configuration as well as the use of multiple and frequently splinted implant units. This resultant primary stability is presumed to prevent any adverse or extensive micromotion at the bone-implant interface. This will in turn avoid the risk of a compromised connective tissue interface that would preclude successful osseointegration. It is also presumed that the laboratory research evidence of more rapid bone ingrowth into the implant surface configuration would also positively influence very early implant stabilization and be a factor in the success of an immediate-loading protocol.

The mechanical stability of the individual implant at the time of surgery has been measured by various techniques. An abundant literature describes the merits and importance of both insertion torque values and resonance frequency analysis, while a number of published articles actually fail to explain how reported implant stability was measured in the first place. The most popular method appears to be the measurement of

> **Box 10-1** Concerns regarding the long-term efficacy and effectiveness of altered loading protocols
>
> - Absence of data on time-dependent clinical outcomes that include heterogeneity of patient age and sex considerations, a variety of selected sites for implant placement, and diverse prosthodontic design prescriptions
> - Evidence that these altered loading protocols provide superior patient satisfaction as well as economic benefits
> - Absence of comparable outcome results for different implant systems

insertion torque values with a stated objective of achieving values in excess of 30 N/cm. While this is a simple method, which suggests that it is clinically useful, it is certainly not an automatic predictor of successful outcome. Since neither method has been shown to be of prognostic value at quantifying the stability of any implant, doubts about the merits of routine use and the relevance of this measurement technique linger.

This chapter reviews relevant and current information associated with altered loading protocols both in diverse bone sites and within the context of the various prosthetic designs required.

## EVOLUTION OF IMMEDIATE AND EARLY LOADING

The early clinical experience with the Brånemark implant system indicated that a 12- to 16-week healing and unloaded phase was necessary for successful osseointegration. It was therefore initially proposed that the implants ideally be submerged during this healing phase. However, certain implant systems challenged this formula, and the elimination of a submerged phase may be regarded as the first step in the move toward early-loading protocols. Within the context of the healing response (see chapter 4), the various loading protocols selected can be categorized as follows:

- Immediate loading: Implants are loaded upon completion of the surgical protocol or the day of surgery.

- Early loading: Implants are loaded one or more days after the first day of surgery, but well in advance of the completion of the interfacial healing phase or osseointegration. Both protocols directly challenge the healing process by introducing loading during wound healing. This means that the notion of an early-loading time frame is a wide and variable one, and therefore not rigorously defined.
- Traditional loading: Implants are not loaded directly, typically for 12 to 16 weeks, as described by different implant system recommendations. This can occur irrespective of whether a stage 2 surgery is planned or not.
- Delayed loading: The healing period is longer than that prescribed for traditional protocols. The major reason for extending the healing period is usually a clinical perception of compromised host site conditions (eg, poor quality bone or grafted sites).

Although a prosthesis may be connected to the implants, they may not be subjected to loading. Initially, occlusal loading may be:

- Absent: Any forces on the implants are generated only through the oral musculature and food bolus via a strategy of diet selection and patient cooperation since healing abutments are in place.
- Partial: The provisional prosthesis is not in occlusion. This approach would apply to partially edentulous patients as opposed to those requiring complete-arch restorations.
- Complete: The prosthesis is in full occlusal contact.

# CLINICAL MANAGEMENT OF PATIENTS

The clinical management of patients to be treated with immediate- or early-loading protocols is identical to that employed for routine implant placement as presented in previous chapters. Some of these points deserve reemphasis:

• The patient's health should not preclude a minor oral surgical procedure, and any brittle systemic condition should be stabilized before implant surgery is undertaken.
• Patients with a history of smoking should be made aware of the inherent risks of their behavior and counseled regarding smoking cessation strategies. While data on the role of cigarette smoking in treatment outcomes with early- or immediate-loading protocols is virtually absent, the negative role of cigarette smoking on the initial healing process, long-term implant survival, and peri-implant bone loss is now well established.
• The residual dentition and supporting periodontal tissues should be healthy prior to initiation of implant treatment. Implant placement and early loading in a mouth with active periodontal disease may be associated with a higher implant failure rate.
• The smile line and its impact on the esthetic result of the proposed treatment should also be addressed. If the proposed implant site is readily visible in the anterior or so-called esthetic zone, the dentist must determine if the site needs to be improved prior to treatment. If this is the case, it would be far more prudent to opt for the traditional loading protocol. To date there is a lack of rigorous scientific evidence supporting simultaneous site augmentation and immediate implant loading.
• All bone sites proposed for implant placement should be assessed radiographically (see chapter 6). A particular technique developed and proposed for immediate-loading protocols promotes the use of additional imaging for treatment planning and simultaneous fabrication of surgical guides and prostheses prior to implant surgery. It remains unclear as to whether this technique is superior to the more traditional imaging protocols in routine use or whether it yields any significant clinical advantage; yet it certainly offers convenience to both patient and dentist. Nonetheless, it comes at an increased economic price for the patient.

The dentist should also discuss the merits of all relevant concerns with the patient and seek to provide answers to the following questions:

• What are the patient's expectations and can they be addressed?
• Is the treatment the most effective one for the patient?
• What are the costs involved, especially if more advanced techniques are planned? Are these additional costs justified?
• Does the patient understand the full implications of treatment, including possible failure?
• Does the dentist have an alternative plan if the proposed treatment plan cannot be executed?

# IMMEDIATE LOADING IN THE EDENTULOUS PATIENT

The anterior area of the mandible, specifically the area between the mental foramina, was the original site selected for studies with both immediate- and early-loading protocols. This seemed like a logical extension of the impressive skills and results that developed from the original management of the edentulous mandible with conventional loading protocols. Published results revealed excellent success rates for immediately loaded implants in this site in both short-term and medium-term studies. Furthermore, radiographic monitoring of peri-implant bone behavior showed marginal bone loss behavior similar to that found after conventional loading protocols, at least within a relatively short-term reporting period.

These results were obtained irrespective of implant type, surface topography (machined or rough-surface implants), and prosthetic designs, which included both fixed and overdenture alternatives. Both approaches have specific considerations pertaining to their prescribed prosthetic designs and are discussed separately.

## Fixed prostheses

Success rates are reported as generally high for implants loaded with fixed prostheses. However, it should be noted that the success rates are lower for short implants (< 7 mm) when they are placed in unfavorable bone morphology and in distal positions. The number of implants prescribed also varied in these studies. Initially a high number of implants were placed, although not always loaded altogether. These studies tended to suggest that implant failures occurred in areas distal to the mental foramina, sites that typically present with compromised bone morphology. More favorable results were reported when fewer implants were placed in the anterior mandible.

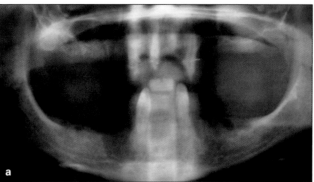

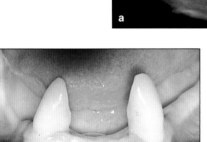

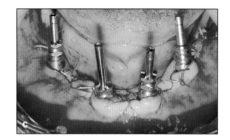

**Fig 10-1** Fixed prosthesis. Panoramic radiograph *(a)* and intraoral view *(b)* of a patient with a terminal dentition. The plan for the mandible is dental extraction and immediate placement and early loading of four implants. The plan for the maxilla includes fabrication of an interim fixed partial denture on the residual dentition, while four implants will be allowed to heal for 4 months. The surgical site is prepared for placement of implants. *(c)* Following positioning, permanent abutments and impression copings are connected to the implants. The provisional tissue-integrated fixed prosthesis *(d)* is inserted in the mandible *(e)*. The interim maxillary fixed partial denture is supported by the residual dentition. *(f)* The final mandibular prosthesis is inserted after healing.

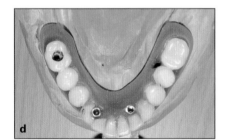

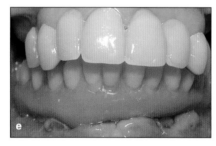

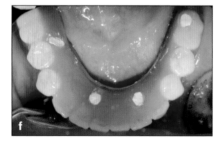

This finding led to numerous studies that investigated the number of implants required to restore the edentulous mandible with a fixed prosthesis. In fact, a few authors reported high success rates using only three implants in the anterior mandible, while other research indicated that loss of one implant in a three-implant system could lead to complete prosthetic failure and necessitate reoperation. This led to the conclusion that rehabilitation of an edentulous patient with three implants is inadvisable and a recommendation that at least four implants be placed in an edentulous mandible to support a multiunit complete-arch prosthesis.

Various techniques may be used to provide patients with a fixed prosthesis (Fig 10-1). Some clinicians opt to convert the existing complete denture or to have a provisional fixed partial denture prepared with adequate relief for abutment connection. Alternatively, provisional or permanent abutments can be attached to the implants, and the denture being worn by the patient at the start of the surgical procedure (or a provisional one) can be hollowed out in the implant sites and connected to the provisional abutment cylinders with autopolymerizing acrylic resin. The denture can then be modified as needed and inserted for immediate functional restoration. If

**Fig 10-2** Mandibular denture that has been converted to an overdenture. Soft tissue remodeling after surgery and bar connection has resulted in loss of the peripheral seal with resultant additional maintenance costs.

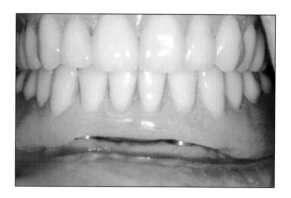

the design choice is a provisional fixed partial denture prepared prior to surgery and with planned necessary relief for abutment connection, it can be used as a surgical guide to facilitate the surgeon's implant positioning. Once desired healing has occurred, fabrication of the final implant-supported fixed partial denture can be undertaken.

A few implant systems actually provide prefabricated frameworks, and implants are inserted in predetermined sites with the help of surgical guides. The same framework can also be used for occlusal relation records. The tooth setup can be verified, and the finished fixed partial denture can then be inserted within a short period of time. A computer-aided prefabricated prosthesis may also be prescribed. However, evidence supporting the superior merits of this technique is sparse, and clinicians should probably approach it cautiously, particularly given the additional costs involved.

The role of the opposing dentition on immediately or early loaded implants is unclear. Published articles have described patients whose opposing dentitions were restored with complete dentures, restored or natural teeth, and implant-supported prostheses. Although reported success rates were high, the specific role of the opposing dentition is yet to be determined conclusively via comparative studies. This suggests that dentists should be careful when managing a patient whose opposing dentition is not a removable prosthesis. In these situations, it appears prudent to avoid loading the implants before some degree of healing has occurred.

Soft tissue behavior around the implants also deserves special consideration. While the literature suggests that it appears to be comparable to that observed with conventional protocols, some researchers have observed soft tissue shrinkage within the first few months after implant placement. This is no different from the soft tissue remodeling observed after conventional surgery; however, it becomes important if it adversely affects the peripheral seal of the prosthesis, especially with an overdenture prosthesis. This concern is probably related to the surgical technique (open flap technique as opposed to punch surgery) and underscores the need for a sufficient period of soft tissue healing to ensure optimal soft tissue health (Fig 10-2).

## Mandibular overdentures

There is convincing evidence supporting immediate- or early-loading protocols for implant-supported and -retained overdentures. It should be recognized, however, that available studies are limited to a very specific site—the mandibular interforaminal area exclusively—and reported high success rates are comparable to those obtained with traditional protocols. Interestingly, short-term studies on early-loading protocols with overdentures even suggest a patient-perceived improvement in denture satisfaction and oral health–related quality of life; however, economic benefits for the patients were not apparent with the selected clinical protocol and recommended modifications. Furthermore, neither implant surface topography nor splinting of the implants was reported as a success determinant. In fact, some studies report successful use of a minimum of two unsplinted machined implants, which suggests that a rough surface and connection or splinting of implants may not be routinely required for mandibular overdenture support.

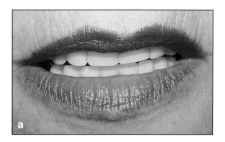
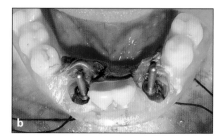

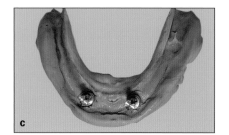
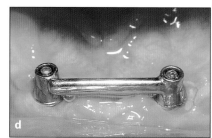

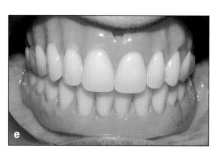

**Fig 10-3** *(a)* Middle-aged patient dissatisfied with a mandibular complete denture because of the lack of stability and retention. Clinical investigation revealed a highly resorbed mandible. *(b)* The plan includes placement of two implants. Because the crest of the ridge is flat, approach is via two punches rather than a full flap. The mandibular denture is used as a surgical guide for implant positioning. *(c)* The mandibular denture was used for a pickup impression of the implants. *(d)* Optimal soft tissue healing is apparent within 5 days. *(e)* The inserted overdenture has addressed the patient's concerns.

The implant overdenture literature underscores the versatility of the technique; three one-stage surgical approaches have been described:

1. Conventional dentures are not worn at all for 1 to 2 weeks or are worn but completely relieved from contact with the obligatory provisional healing abutments on the implants. Eventually, a tissue conditioner is used to optimize the fit of the provisional prosthesis for the duration of the selected healing phase. The clinical premise is that the time-dependent resiliency of the tissue conditioners employed will attenuate some of the occlusal stresses transmitted to the healing interface without disturbing its progress. A definitive prosthesis is fabricated and connected via the selected abutments and attachments at a later stage, and within a time frame of 3 to 4 months after implant surgery.

2. Dentures are not worn for 2 weeks or are relined and inserted immediately after the first surgical stage and placement of suitably long healing abutments. Final retentive components are connected within 3 weeks and following healing of the soft tissues. The definitive prosthesis directly loads the implants and challenges the osseointegration process early on, but perhaps to a greater extent than in the first technique.

3. Retentive attachments (typically a bar and clip assembly) are provided within the first few days postsurgically, and the final prosthesis is inserted as soon as possible.

Clear evidence endorses the assumption that a relined denture can be worn the same day implants are inserted. The decision as to when to proceed with the final prosthesis will then depend on the surgical protocol employed. If the surgery included a full flap, it is recommended that fabrication of the prosthesis wait for soft tissue healing. Conversely if surgery was very conservative, for example, a punch technique, fabrication of the final prosthesis can be undertaken at the dentist's discretion (Fig 10-3).

## Maxillary prostheses

Success rates for immediately loaded maxillary implants are lower than those for the mandible and also limited to the anterior zone between the maxillary sinuses. These results should be viewed with caution because published reports are limited as a result of restricted numbers of patients, grouping of completely and partially edentulous patients, and relatively short observation periods. Furthermore, reported results are mainly for fixed prostheses. There is therefore limited information to support the routine use of overdentures with such protocols in the edentulous maxilla.

Unlike in the mandible, in the edentulous maxilla the minimum number of implants required with these protocols is not clear cut. Because the edentulous maxilla tends to have softer or poorer quality bone than the mandible, authors have suggested that more implants are required, sometimes up to 12 implants. On the other hand, there is limited evidence that patients can be treated successfully with a conventional number of implants (five or six). This suggests similarities of outcome for both protocols and precludes the need for additional implants.

Some reports are quite optimistic about the use of rough-surfaced implants in sites with soft bone conditions like those encountered in the maxilla and speculate that this would be advantageous because of the promotion of faster healing. However, the literature does not fully support this contention for the edentulous maxilla. In some comparative short-term case series, roughened implants performed better than machine-turned ones; other studies reported successful outcomes if machine-turned implants were placed in the anterior maxilla with alterations in the surgical method. These success outcomes must be interpreted within the context of the study design. It certainly underscores the need for more clinical research to better understand if modified implant surface topography plays a clinically significant role in the success of these protocols.

An overall provisional conclusion is that caution is indicated in the management of the edentulous maxilla with immediate- or early-loading protocols. It should also be emphasized that clinical researchers who have reported successful outcomes with the edentulous maxilla are highly experienced. Consequently, their results should not be interpreted as proof that their described protocols can be used routinely.

Nonetheless, a number of recent publications suggest optimism for early-loading protocols, even in the maxilla. One particularly interesting example is the recently described Columbus Bridge Protocol, which combines specific surgical and prosthodontic procedures to manufacture a screw-retained maxillary full-arch provisional partial denture and which permits early loading in patients with a residual dentition. The surgery is performed in native bone and through fresh sockets without any form of site improvement. Its objective is the placement of four to six external hexagon implants in the anterior maxillary zone between the mesial bilateral boundaries of the maxillary sinuses. This surgical placement protocol requires torque measurements ≥ 40 N/cm for all the implants, with the two distalmost having inclinations tangential to the anterior sinus walls, allowing them to be 13 to 18 mm in length. (This is in contrast to much shorter implants otherwise placed in their long axes in these specific anatomic sites). Two to four anterior implants are inserted in the lateral incisor-canine zone as predetermined by a customized surgical guide so as to complete the objective of optimized potential abutment support. Straight or pre-angled conical abutments are used to compensate for the resultant diversities in implant inclinations. Traditional clinical prosthodontic stages—impression and jaw registrations—lead to the fabrication of a provisional screw-retained fixed prosthesis, which is luted onto the nonhexed conical abutment cylinders by a dual composite cement some 24 hours later. This completes the initial phase of providing a passive fit for a prosthesis design that includes the following: no distal cantilevers, acrylic resin occlusal surfaces, and a palladium-alloy framework to increase strength and rigidity.

The preliminary report included 29 patients with 38 implants and a recorded 93.5% implant cumulative survival rate at 24 months. Nine implants failed during the first 3 months. The mean bone levels were 0.84 and 0.96 mm below the reference point (implant-abutment junction) at the 1- and 2-year follow-up appointments, respectively. No significant differences were noted between upright and angulated implants nor between implants placed in healed bone versus extraction sockets. Figure 10-4 presents a case from the study.

The limitations of this short-term follow-up study certainly preclude definitive conclusions. Other similar studies also lacked a control group, patient randomization, and patient-mediated outcome measures. However, much promise has been attributed to the notion that patients with a dentate maxilla can be rendered edentulous and rehabilitated virtually immediately with fixed prostheses with negligible morbidity and without expensive computer-guided surgical options. This sort of preliminary research may be the harbinger of what scrupulous and traditional protocols can yield in the search for predictable treatment outcomes with an early-loading management strategy.

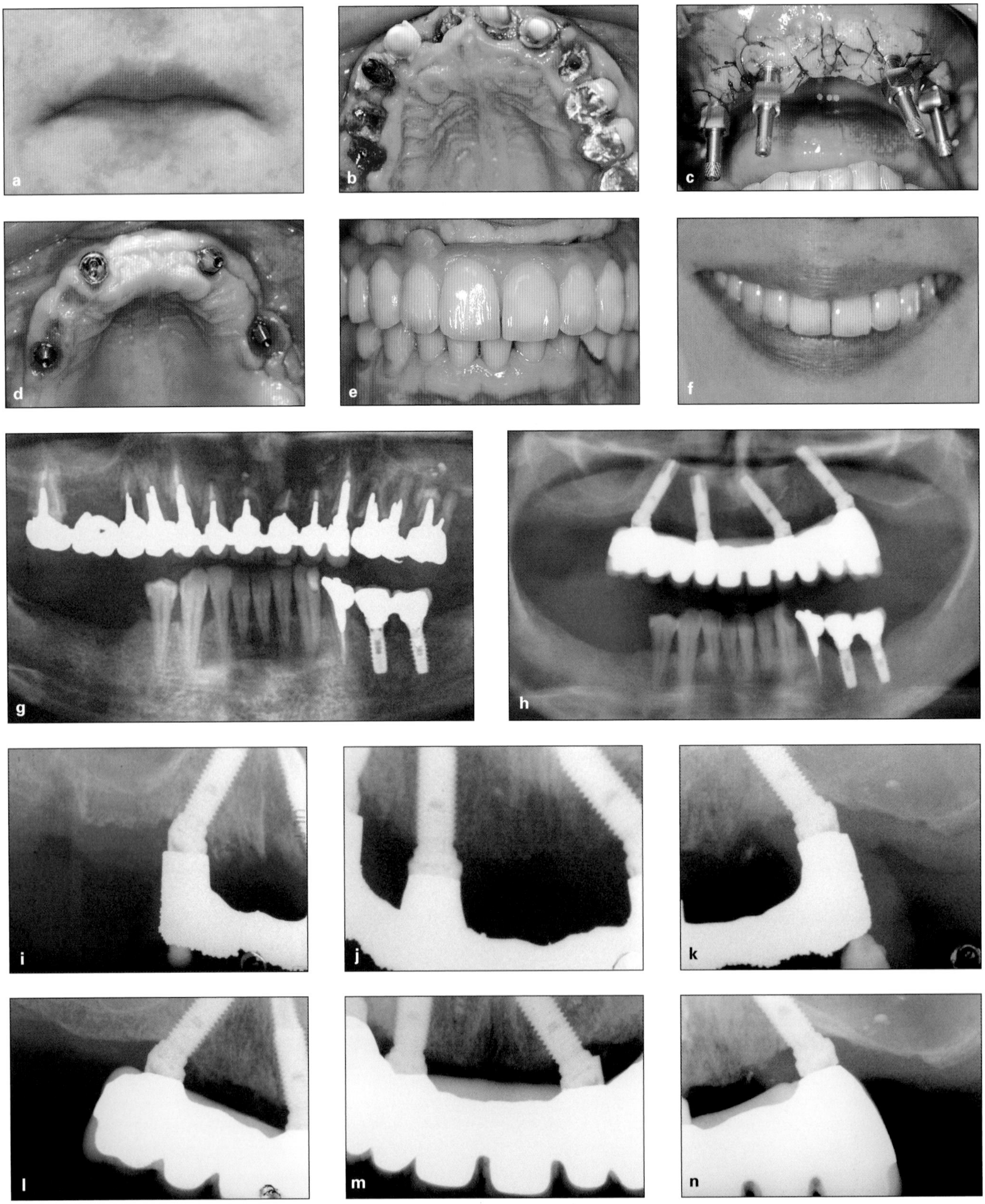

**Fig 10-4** Facial (a) and maxillary occlusal (b) views of a 42-year-old female patient with severely neglected oral health. (c) Implants and impression copings are in place with completion of soft tissue suturing. (d) Occlusal view of healed soft tissues after 4 months. (e and f) The esthetic result with fixed prosthesis in place. (g) Presurgical panoramic radiograph. (h) Panoramic radiograph 24 hours postsurgery. (i to k) Radiographs of implants 4 months postsurgery. (l to n) Radiographs of implants after 3 years of functional loading.

# Immediate Loading in the Partially Edentulous Patient

## Multiple-tooth replacement

The partially edentulous patient may have single or multiple edentulous sites. Due consideration should be given to the length of the edentulous span, its position in the arch, and whether the span is tooth bound or an unbounded distal extension. A tooth-bound edentulous site that is in the anterior zone can be approached in the same way as a fully edentulous arch. However, if the edentulous span is in a posterior site, such as a Kennedy Class I or II partially edentulous maxilla or mandible, the dentist should be particularly cautious because the zones typically include compromised bone. This may therefore preclude an immediate-loading protocol or early-loading protocol and should be discussed beforehand with the patient.

If the edentulous site is tooth bound, the implants can be restored and, to some extent, enjoy organized loading protection from the adjacent teeth during both functional and parafunctional excursive movements. When the implants are in a distal position, the loading potential of the implants and the residual dentition must be reconciled and, if possible, the excursive occlusal contacts should be on the natural teeth.

Research supporting the use of immediate loading and early loading in the partially edentulous patient is limited and does not permit any compelling conclusions. Although various clinical reports have been published, the research designs have various shortcomings, such as a restricted number of patients, grouping of different types of prostheses and edentulous sites, lack of standardization, use of different implants, and short follow-up periods. However, a one-stage approach has been definitively and successfully used and can be safely recommended when the surgical procedure is routine. On the other hand, whenever additional surgery is required, such as concomitant bone augmentation along with implant placement, it is recommended that the implants be permitted a submerged healing phase.

The type of implant surface employed also deserves special consideration within the context of the partially edentulous patient. Studies suggest that when the bone quality is favorable (type 2 or 3), good results can be obtained with any implant surface. In fact, a number of authors have reported that successful osseointegration can also be obtained with machine-turned implants used together with a modified surgical approach that seeks to establish primary stability (Box 10-2).

**Box 10-2** SURGICAL MODIFICATIONS FOR IMPLANT PLACEMENT IN TYPE 4 BONE

- Avoidance of bone tapping
- Avoidance of countersinking
- Underpreparation of the osteotomy site
- Use of narrower drills
- Site preparation with osteotomes
- Attainment of bicortical stabilization
- Use of a wider implant when the original implant diameter does not achieve the desired stability

In poor-quality bone sites (type 4), the body of evidence suggests that a modified implant surface actually may be preferable. Furthermore, it has been shown that immediate- and early-loading protocols should be avoided in patients who exhibit bruxism because a higher failure rate was reported for this particular group. However, these observations are largely anecdotal and underscore the need for long-term clinical trials to rigorously ascertain the viability of these preliminary clinical findings.

## Single-tooth replacement

Various studies on the immediate loading of single-tooth–supported prostheses have reported success rates comparable to those achieved with a conventional loading protocol. Implants have been placed in all sites of both arches for this purpose. The single-tooth prosthesis lends itself well to these protocols, because it can be protected from the risk of adverse occlusal contacts by the adjacent teeth. Moreover, the implant can be restored at chairside with the use of provisional abutments and readily available materials that are used routinely in conventional crown and prosthesis fabrication (Fig 10-5).

The role of bone quality in the success of single-tooth prostheses is not clear. Conflicting results have been observed and reported in so-called soft (type 4) bone, making it imprudent to provide immediate restoration of an implant placed in bone with these exhibited low values of stability. A safer approach would be to wait for the necessary bone healing to occur. Irrespective of the bone quality described, the marginal bone loss around single implants is reported as being of the same magnitude as described previously with a conventional approach, at least in short- to medium-term studies.

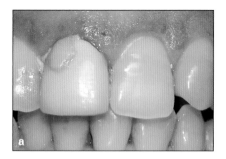 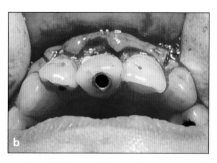 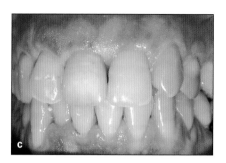

**Fig 10-5** Immediate loading of a single-implant prosthesis. *(a)* The middle-aged patient has a failed porcelain-fused-to-metal crown. Radiographic imaging has indicated the presence of a subgingival fracture. *(b)* A flap is raised, and the fractured root is extracted with forceps. An implant is placed immediately and restored with a provisional crown. *(c)* Following 2 months of soft tissue healing, the interim crown is replaced with the permanent prosthesis.

The effect of occlusion on immediately restored single-implant prostheses is not entirely clear. High success rates are reported when restorations are placed in complete occlusal contact, but other authors have also described a lower success rate when restorations were in complete functional loading or even in light occlusal contact. Further studies are required to conclusively determine the role of occlusion in these clinical situations. Keeping the provisional prosthesis out of occlusion may very well be a prudent strategy since it is presumed to permit the implant to osseointegrate in an unloaded fashion.

As discussed previously for the management of the edentulous maxilla, the data supporting immediate- and early-loading protocols of single- and multiple-tooth prostheses in the partially edentulous patients are the outgrowth of only short-term clinical studies presented by skilled clinicians. Therefore, the results cannot be taken as proof that these protocols can be routinely used in clinical practice. Caution is necessary in both proper case selection and implementation of these protocols.

## IMMEDIATE IMPLANT PLACEMENT

Proposed and popularly accepted advantages for placing implants in fresh extraction sockets include the preservation of bone, soft tissue anatomy, and esthetics—the so-called emergence profile (Fig 10-6). It has also been theorized that treatment time and associated costs can be reduced by avoiding an intermediate bone-healing stage with the associated need for an interim prosthesis. Strong evidence for this method is still unavailable, and published reports are of short duration and limited in numbers. Additionally, in certain reports the extraction sockets were not used as implant sites but were obliterated because of surgical reduction of the residual ridge. Caution is essential when the clinician embarks on protocols involving immediate placement of implants in extraction sites. Clinical researchers have shown that success per se was not compromised by placement in extraction sockets as long as primary stability was achieved. Yet, recorded success rates were unpredictable when implants were placed in morphologically compromised jawbone sites, including some with a history of previous periodontal disease.

Single-tooth prostheses have been placed in both fresh extraction sockets and healed sites. Reported reasons for tooth extraction include unresolved infection, tooth trauma, retained root portions, unrestorable crowns, and root resorption. Placement and immediate or early loading of an implant in a fresh extraction site compromised by the presence of infection is not recommended, and the literature reports a lower success rate in these situations. The placement of implants in fresh extraction sites should be avoided in clinical situations with on-

**Fig 10-6** Immediate loading of a single-implant prosthesis using flapless surgery. *(a)* An elderly patient has a fractured lateral incisor. The plan is for extraction of the root stump *(b)* and immediate placement and restoration of an implant *(c)*. *(d)* Following adequate soft tissue healing, the final prosthesis is inserted.

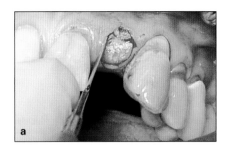
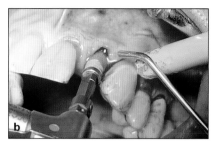
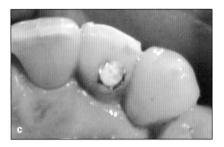
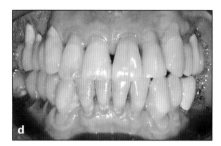

going inflammatory processes such as active periodontal and periapical infection.

The initial surgical step is the careful removal of the tooth so that the walls of the bony socket are preserved. The socket is then assessed to make sure it is clear of infection. The clinician should then decide on where the implant will be placed. In the case of an anterior tooth, the implant is placed in the available socket. However, if the tooth is a posterior one with more than one root, a socket site that will give the implant the necessary primary stability must be selected or prepared. In the case of a posterior maxillary tooth, this would probably mean the palatal socket; both mesial and distal sockets can be used to replace a mandibular molar.

Site preparation usually follows the specific implant manufacturer's guidelines, although the clinician should consider underpreparing the site to preserve local bone anatomy and improve the primary stability of the implant. If the necessary stability is achieved, the implant can be restored with a provisional prosthesis. In the event that the implant does not have adequate stability, the implant should not be loaded but allowed to heal unhindered.

Management of the defect between the implant and socket must be considered; some form of grafting is the usual approach. Researchers have reported the use of autogenous bone harvested from the implant osteotomy sites as well as

xenografts and, in some patients, no material was grafted in the defects (see chapter 7). Some of these protocols are still being researched, and strong clinical evidence is still lacking. Indeed no single technique has been proven superior for bone augmentation around implants placed in fresh extraction sockets. A recent systematic review on the efficacy and effectiveness of barrier membranes concluded that further evidence is needed to determine whether such membranes prevent bone resorption in autologous onlay bone grafts; it is clear that further long-term clinical research is required to support most of the currently applied interventions.

A presumed major advantage for immediate restoration of an extracted tooth is the preservation of the surrounding soft tissues, specifically the gingival and interdental papilla. This can provide a highly esthetic result because of the presence of the crown during the healing phase. It is recommended that a provisional crown be used during the healing phase before a definitive crown is fabricated. The use of a provisional crown permits modification of the soft tissue profile by adding or reducing prosthetic material until the desired soft tissue profile is achieved. This same provisional crown can then be used as an impression coping, providing the dental technician with an impression of the healed surrounding soft tissues and the position of the desired definitive crown.

## Conclusion

Generally speaking, immediate and early loading of implants may be regarded as safe procedures. However, there are two important caveats that must be considered:

1. Most published reports are of short-term duration and lack methodologic rigor.
2. Reported treatment outcomes are largely implant based and rarely address patient-mediated concerns.

Nonetheless, a number of prudent conclusions can be reached, and they provide suitable guidelines for clinicians and patients:

1. The anterior mandible provides the most predictable results with both fixed and overdenture prostheses and should be the first site of choice for application of these modified protocols. Implant design and surface topography do not appear to influence success rates in this site. It is advisable to place at least four implants in the edentulous anterior mandible to support a multiunit fixed prosthesis.
2. Emerging evidence suggests that reasonable success rates are also achievable for the anterior maxilla. However, these optimistic reports should be approached with caution given the poor bone quality frequently encountered in this area and the need for excellent surgical operating skills.
3. Proper site selection, appropriate imaging, scrupulous surgical judgment, and, where indicated, modification of surgical technique are necessary for the execution of these protocols, especially in posterior zones (Class I or II partial edentulism).
4. The single-tooth prosthesis is indicated in sites where immediate, predictable implant stability can be achieved. Implant placement in extraction sites should be restricted to those sites without a history of infection.

Patients and dentists are vulnerable to industry-initiated information that proposes techniques and treatment schedules that claim more efficacious and immediate solutions for dental replacement needs. Generalized information spread by word of mouth as well as the Internet is readily available for all, including patients who demand such protocols from their clinicians. It has therefore become imperative that the dentist critically review information sources along with clinical published reports before offering new treatment protocols. Patients should also be made aware that general information on certain techniques may not automatically apply to their specific dental needs. The fact that early-loading protocols are proposed as a virtual panacea must still be reconciled with a scientific understanding of time-dependent bone and soft tissue healing processes.

## Recommended Reading

Attard NJ, Zarb GA. Immediate and early implant loading protocols: A literature review of clinical studies. J Prosthet Dent 2005;94:242–258.

DeLuca S, Habsha E, Zarb GA. The effect of smoking on osseointegrated dental implants. 1. Implant survival. Int J Prosthodont 2006;19:482–489.

DeLuca S, Zarb GA. The effect of smoking on osseointegrated dental implants. 2. Peri-implant bone loss. Int J Prosthodont 2006;19:560–566.

Elsubeihi ES, Zarb G. Implant prosthodontics in medically compromised challenged patients: The University of Toronto experience. J Can Dent Assoc 2002;68:103–108.

Esposito M, Grusovin MG, Worthington HV, Coulthard P. Interventions for replacing missing teeth: Bone augmentation techniques for dental implant treatment. Cochrane Database Syst Rev 2006 Jan 25;(1):CD003607.

Gielkens PF, Bos RR, Raghoebar GM, Stegenga B. Is there evidence that barrier membranes prevent bone resorption in autologous bone grafts during the healing period? A systematic review. Int J Oral Maxillofac Implants 2007;22:390–398.

Szmukler-Moncler S, Salama H, Reingewirtz Y, Dubruille J. Timing of loading and effect of micromotion on bone-dental implant interface: Review of experimental literature. J Biomed Mater Res 1998;43:192–203.

# Osseointegration Failure

### David Chvartszaid | Sreenivas Koka | George A. Zarb

Popular acceptance of implant therapy by both the general public and dental profession has reinforced the perception that prosthetic abutments, whether teeth or implants, may be regarded as equivalent to one another. Consequently, if a particular clinical situation does not permit natural tooth support for a fixed prosthesis, an implant-supported one is frequently accepted as a close second or, perhaps, even better alternative. This perception is certainly reinforced (with documented justification) by today's professional mantra that "implants are better than natural teeth."

The objectives of complication-free treatment and successful osseointegration are not always achieved. This is a realistic reminder that surgical interventions may elicit unpredictable healing responses, while prosthodontic ones introduce inherent outcome risks. It is, therefore, prudent to recognize that a combination of both interventions via implant-supported prostheses may yield treatment complications or treatment failures, particularly when osseointegration is compromised. Unexpected and adverse outcomes in implant dentistry often result from lapses in treatment planning or clinical judgment: improper patient or site selection; incorrect selection of number, size, and location of implants; implant malalignment; poor prosthetic design; or incorrect selection of implant type. These errors frequently result in mechanical failures or complications at the level of the prosthesis or the supporting components. Fortunately, these compromised situations may be salvageable, although they invariably challenge prosthodontic ingenuity in the process. They are also largely avoidable, if established protocols are scrupulously followed.

Biologic failures occur when one or more implants either do not osseointegrate or else fail to maintain a state of osseointegration. The ultimate seriousness of either event depends on whether or not the prescribed prosthesis-supporting role becomes compromised. For example, there is a significant treatment outcome difference between failed osseointegration in a single-tooth replacement and a similar occurrence in a multi-implant–supported prosthesis for an edentulous patient. Multi-implant–supported prostheses are often designed with potential complications in mind and may continue functioning despite the loss of one of the implants.

It should be pointed out that the dental profession may be unduly harsh on itself when such events are encountered. Orthopedic literature, for example, speaks of the need for treatment *revisions* (rather than treatment *failure*) when time-dependent loosened hip implant failure occurs. Dental clinicians must accept that implant-dependent interventions have finite life spans and that *maintenance* and *revision* are terms more applicable to treatment planning conversations with patients than terms such as *complication* and *failure*. Simply put, many of the factors necessary for successful implant therapy are beyond the clinician's control.

When implant failure occurs, some dentists presume that the pathogenesis of tooth loss and implant loss are identical, with concepts of disease activity and prosthesis failure that apply to natural teeth transposed on their implant replacements. It is sometimes said that, logically, implant failure must be bacterially induced and similar to periodontitis, yielding the posttransposition term *peri-implantitis*. In addition, the unpredictable frequency, duration, and magnitude of parafunctional occlusal forces have also been shown to impact the longevity of fixed and removable restorations supported by natural teeth. Consequently, another large constituency of practitioners presume that implant failures result from a disparity between implants' holding power (ie, the amount and quality of osseointegrated response) and occlusal loading. Thus, the proposed concepts of infection-induced implant failure and occlusal adverse load–induced implant failure have received the most attention when causes of implant failure are discussed.

## ATTACHMENT DIFFERENCES

Before implant infection and occlusal adverse loading are reviewed as precursors or causes of implant failure, a reminder of the salient similarities and differences between teeth and implants takes precedence. Implants are frequently described as *tooth root analogs*; yet the genesis and specific nature of their interfacial attachments to host bone differ. These differences are subtle but profound in many ways, and their analysis may help highlight the differences in disease initiation and progression.

To begin with, the tooth attachment mechanism results from a developmental process driven by genetic influences. Implants, by contrast, are the result of planned surgical site preparation that is obturated with an alloplastic material and that hopefully results in a controlled healing response. Attachment to epithelium, soft connective tissue, and bone—three host tissues extending from the occlusal to the apical direction—may or may not occur. The preponderance of current knowledge regarding the interface of implants and host tissues comes from studies with machined commercially pure titanium implant surfaces. Epithelium appears to attach to such surfaces in a manner somewhat similar as it does to teeth, resulting in a mechanically fragile surface adhesion rather than true attachment.

However, the other two tissues clearly do not mimic nature. Soft connective tissue fibers are unable to attach to implant surfaces in the manner that Sharpey fibers attach to cementum covering root surfaces. The result is merely an abutting of soft scarlike connective tissue against the implant surface. A tooth is attached to the surrounding bone by means of an intermediary tissue, the periodontal ligament. A healthy periodontal ligament permits very slight, transient tooth movement in response to intermittent heavy occlusal stresses, as well as orthodontic tooth movement in response to light controlled forces. It can also permit varying degrees of mobility in the presence of periodontal ligament inflammation or widening and in situations of compromised attachment support. The periodontal ligament may be vulnerable to the host inflammatory response to virulence factors associated with pathogenic organisms in dental plaque, and this vulnerability may manifest as progressive crestal alveolar bone loss.

Implants, on the other hand, are secured to bone by the osseointegrated interface, which, as stated in chapter 2, appears to be a direct fusion of bone into the microporosities and macroporosities on the implant surface. The resilience of bone means that implants are significantly less mobile than teeth surrounded by a periodontal ligament. Indeed, osseointegrated implants are clinically immobile.

The induced interfacial response results from a controlled recruitment of those determinants of bone healing consequent to application of a specific and repeatable surgical protocol. The osteotomy site of precisely prepared, and perhaps injured, bone is plugged by an implant to achieve primary stability. The ensuing ankylosis-generating interfacial response represents tissue maturation through new bone growth (modeling) and subsequent turnover (remodeling). Peri-implant inflammatory changes of gingiva or bone that mimic changes caused by periodontal disease are occasionally observed. However, the progression to any resultant loss of osseointegration is rare, and its pathogenesis is incompletely understood and is thought to be governed by a different set of etiologic factors from those determining periodontal tissue destruction around teeth. Recognition of this fundamental interfacial difference—developmental phenomenon versus induced healing response—permits a more prudent interpretation of why implant failure may occur and how it may be prevented.

## CAUSES OF IMPLANT FAILURE

### The infection theory

The first patients treated with implants were fully edentulous, frequently prosthetically maladaptive, long-term complete denture–wearers. Reliable information as to why these patients had lost their teeth was unavailable. Although the causes of edentulism tend to be cultural and socioeconomic and not exclusively disease related, it is reasonable to surmise that a substantial number of patients from the early Gothenburg and Toronto studies endured prior periodontal disease. This presumption is reinforced by the observation that the recorded residual ridge reductions in these patients were very similar to those recorded in edentulous patients with confirmed histories of total tooth loss from advanced periodontal disease.

The impressive successful outcomes demonstrated in these early studies were accompanied by a virtual absence of recordable gingival morbidity. This led to the classification of all associated adverse gingival observations as nuisance side effects, akin more to sores from denture irritation than to a periodontally inspired process.

Dentists who were skeptical of implants' initial success attributed the high success of osseointegration in completely edentulous patients to a changed bacterial ecology of the oral cavity. They reasoned that the absence of teeth led to absence of periodontal pathogens. However, their forecast for managing partially edentulous patients with implants was an ominous one: They expected that pathogens present around natural teeth would "seed" the pockets around implants and pose a risk for eventual implant failure.

The isolation of periodontal pathogens from sites around failing implants was cited as sufficient confirmation of the infection theory of osseointegration failure. It extended the notion that residual periodontal pockets around remaining teeth provide niches of infection for adjacent implants that will compromise an implant's otherwise healthy attachment mechanism. The observation of suppuration around some failed implants lent further credence to this theory. Inevitable questions were posed:

- Is the reason for tooth loss an important predictor of implant treatment outcomes?
- Can successful implants maintain their attachment in patients with periodontal disease?
- Will implants survive better than the teeth they are meant to replace, or are we merely substituting one problem for another?

It was not long before numerous reports sought to address and clarify such concerns as they questioned the basis or conclusions of the infection theory of implant failure. Both controlled and uncontrolled studies convincingly described an apparent lack of impact of periodontal disease and periodontal disease parameters on implant treatment and success. Certainly, bacteria are isolated from around implants; yet no consistent pathogenic flora is observed in patients, irrespective of a previous history of periodontal disease.

It appears that most of the literature on susceptibility of implants to periodontitis-like processes ultimately stems from "ligature studies" in experimental animals and from isolation of periodontal pathogens around failed implants in humans. However, ligature studies do not accurately represent the etiology and progression of peri-implant bone destruction in humans, and their findings lack corroboration from human studies. As such, their scientific worth is questionable. The detection of some bacterial species at sites of failed implants does not suggest cause and effect; there is a risk of confusing etiology of failure with the consequence of the asymptomatic failed implant remaining in the mouth (possibly months or even years) until its detection. Are the bacteria detected at sites of failed implants the primary cause of the failure or do they merely represent secondary opportunistic colonization? Since failed implants that remain in the mouth until their detection are surrounded by a soft tissue capsule that does not attach to the implant, this potential deep space (the length of the implant) can be readily secondarily colonized by a variety of bacteria.

Attention should also be drawn to the observation that periodontally compromised teeth that are retained and treated tend not to adversely affect the status of adjacent teeth, while retention of periodontally compromised teeth without treatment has a destructive effect on adjacent teeth.

Furthermore, the association between periodontal disease and osseointegration loss does not appear to be epidemiologically compelling. Implants in partially edentulous patients perform as well as, and according to some reports even better than, those in completely edentulous patients (failure rates: complete edentulism, 7%; partial edentulism, 4%; single tooth, 2%). If bacterial conditions affecting remaining teeth had a significant negative impact on the success of implants within the same mouth, implants in completely edentulous patients should have significantly better success rates. However, this is clearly not the case. Thus, the presence of natural teeth (and their associated bacterial flora) has no negative impact on the incidence of implant failure or complications.

Patterns of implant failure over time are also not consistent with periodontal disease history as a contributing factor. Uncontrolled periodontal disease progression leads to cumulative bone loss over time and a resultant progressive tooth loss in subjects with untreated periodontitis. Yet, patterns of implant failure documented in long-term epidemiologic studies demonstrate that the incidence of osseointegration failure occurs within a relatively short period of time following the surgical placement (typically, within first 2 years). So-called late failures, or subsequent implant losses, appear to be negligible. When late failures are observed in significant numbers, these can often be traced to wear and tear of poorly designed prosthodontic components (as was seen with the original IMZ system [Friadent]) or disintegration of fixture surface coating (as was seen with some early hydroxyapatite coatings).

Some studies suggest an association between periodontal diseases and implant failure. There are reasons to believe that this apparent association is due to the confounding effect of smoking and other factors (eg, uncontrolled diabetes) that negatively affect both conditions. Smoking is a risk factor for periodontal disease and poor periodontal treatment prognosis. At the same time, smoking is a known risk factor for implant failure. Factors that affect wound healing and incidence of postoperative infection (eg, uncontrolled diabetes) also affect both periodontal disease and implant failure. Therefore, the association of periodontal disease and implant failure in some epidemiologic studies may be attributed to inadequate control for underlying etiologic factors (eg, smoking and diabetes) and should be looked at with suspicion.

Differences in the bone attachment mechanisms of teeth and implants demand a different explanation for the pathogeneses of periodontal disease and osseointegration loss. Plaque accumulation around teeth is a compelling etiologic agent in periodontitis, and current clinical concepts in periodontal infection control emphasize the significance of prevention of bacterial plaque accumulations via oral hygiene protocols. In fact, the long-term success of managing periodontitis-susceptible patients is based on the introduction of measures that provide the patients with support for their own efforts to control the infection. Consequently, a schedule of regular monitoring recall visits that aim at providing supportive care completes the current therapeutic formula.

A subject-specific threshold level of bacterial overload also appears to exist that influences both management and outcome of the infection. Hence, host-related systemic, behavioral, and environmental factors must be taken into account, over and above the presence of an adverse biofilm. Furthermore, much current research is directed toward identification of both subject- and tooth site–associated factors that predict treatment outcomes.

Plaque accumulation around implants can certainly lead to superficial inflammatory changes. Therefore, design features of implants should aim to eliminate plaque-retentive surfaces. The development of rough surface implants is driven by the desire to promote osseous healing. Unfortunately, should the surface become inadvertently exposed to the oral cavity, the same rough surfaces are easily contaminated by plaque and also uneasily decontaminated.

Deep soft tissue pockets that result from the presence of thick areas of gingival tissues over the implant bony site may also act as nuisance sites in the context of easy and uneventful management of plaque accumulation. However, the presence of peri-implant gingivitis (mucositis) is largely inconsequential and does not appear to automatically progress to peri-implant bone loss. Such a progression has most certainly not been demonstrated in human studies. Nonetheless, some studies found slight additional implant bone loss over long observation periods in patients with histories of either poor oral hygiene (specifically, in the anterior mandible) or smoking.

A rigid insistence on a periodontitis-like pathogenicity for implant failure has even led to therapeutic initiatives for treating failing or ailing implants—a regrettable attempt to apply periodontal disease treatment protocols to the management of compromised osseointegration. The literature on the subject reveals numerous shortcomings, and the lack of human clinical studies that have sufficient scientific rigor to address the role of oral bacteria in implant failure leaves the dental profession with believers and disbelievers pitted against each other to debate whether bacterially induced infection is a primary cause of implant failure. The role of dental plaque in eliciting soft tissue inflammation is readily acknowledged. However, we believe that the compelling weight of circumstantial evidence shows that in most cases of implant failure, bacterially induced infection is neither the cause nor a cofactor.

At the end of the day, a prudent interpretation of the available literature and our own clinical experiences permit the following conclusions:

1. The premise of the infection theory of implant failure underscored the importance of periodontal treatment of any residual dentition prior to implant placement and the importance of routine oral hygiene maintenance. The latter objective remains a laudatory one because any surgical intervention benefits from an uncontaminated field of operation.
2. Patients with a history of periodontal disease without active sites of infection are most certainly candidates for implant treatment, and no increased risk of implant failure should be expected. Because good oral hygiene practices are expected and demanded of all patients, no special recall regimens are needed beyond what would be normally prescribed for maintaining routine oral health.
3. An increase in the vulnerability of coronal bone levels to pathogenic microorganisms may indeed occur as a result of long-term cervical exposure of the currently popular rough implant surfaces. This remains a concern in the context of an understanding of cervical bone level behavior in different bone quality sites under different loading and behavioral scenarios.

Implant failures are discovered when submerged implants are uncovered surgically. Clearly such implants have not been exposed to oral flora for months, and the discovery of failure is usually accompanied by a striking lack of signs of infection. For this reason alone, it is prudent to acknowledge that many implant failures result from means other than infection, plaque induced or otherwise.

## The occlusal adverse load theory

Biomechanical adverse loading at the bone-implant interface has been hypothesized to cause, or contribute to, loss of osseointegration as a result of marginal bone loss or induction of a fibrous connective tissue interface. The theory is suggested by clinical, animal, and finite-element analysis studies. The basic premise is that loading of implants leads to micromotion at the bone-implant interface and a transfer of forces to the adjacent bone. The amount of force transferred depends on many variables, including the degree or quality of osseointegration, the geometry and surface characteristics of the implant, and the quality and quantity of host bone.

While some strain at the implant-bone interface is regarded as desirable, unfavorable strains beyond a certain threshold can produce deformation of the bone and an uncontrolled biologic response with a gradually resultant implant loosening. Adverse load forces are multidimensional in nature and affected by numerous presumed sources, such as parafunctional tooth contact activities, the number and distribution of implants employed for prosthesis support, the type and possible misfit of the framework, and cantilever lengths.

Biomechanical forces can be classified as either compressive, shear, or tensile. Axially directed compressive and tensile forces are generally regarded as more favorable than shear ones. The resulting load type at the interface can be either static (eg, arising from continuous application of low loads such as from a poorly fitting framework) or dynamic (eg, a repeated application of a parafunctional occlusal load). Research has clearly demonstrated that bone appears to have a relatively high tolerance against static forces. Hence, it is now readily accepted that implants can be used for orthodontic anchorage, and the once suspected negative impact of prosthesis misfit on the maintenance of osseointegration has not been shown to be a clinically relevant phenomenon.

Bone does not remain in a static and unchanged state, but instead actively responds to the forces of the external environment by altering its internal architecture. Mechanical forces on bone can induce it to undergo cellular changes and result in bone remodeling. Mechanical fatigue damage (microdamage) constantly occurs in bone, and remodeling can usually repair the damage and keep it from accumulating. Thus, the damaged bone is removed and replaced with new bone.

Adverse loading the bone can increase the microdamage, overwhelming the normal bony maintenance mechanisms. The damaged bone is not remodeled fast enough to keep up with accumulated damage. In the pathologic adverse load zone, the strain levels are beyond the ability of the bone to repair itself, leading to microfractures and net loss of bone and potentially resulting in dental implant failure. It has also been speculated that bone quality deteriorates near sites subjected to increased bone turnover from adverse loading. However, it should be pointed out that there are also many host-related factors affecting bone quality and volume.

Finite Element Analysis (FEA) is a computerized investigative method that uses a mathematical model to determine the mechanical stress arising in various objects and their environment as a result of forces affecting the system. This technique has been utilized to predict strain distribution around implants under various loading scenarios. Finite element analysis studies have shown that peak stresses and strains occur at the most occlusal crestal point on the cortical bone around dental implants. In general, computer simulations tend to support the concept that it is possible for excessive external forces on dental prostheses to cause unfavorable osseous changes around implants retaining them and ultimately result in implant failure.

However, despite the abundance of circumstantial evidence, direct undisputed clinical evidence for this hypothesis is lacking. Finite element analyses are useful for generating hypotheses and testing our basic biomechanical mechanisms, but the mul-

tiple assumptions they make need to be clinically validated, and their predictions need to be corroborated by hard clinical data generated in long-term prospective studies. Animal studies are difficult to compare with each other or with the human scenario they are meant to emulate. The available estimates of maximum biting forces in commonly used laboratory animal experiments; the known rates of healing in animals; and animal jaw anatomy, physiology, and biomechanics all differ substantially from the clinical situation in humans. Thus, extrapolating data from animal experiments to the human model is problematic. The lack of congruence is likely responsible for the largely contradictory evidence thus far obtained from animal studies. Clinical human studies are equally difficult to conduct because of the presence of confounding variables and difficulties in precisely measuring and standardizing cumulative occlusal loading vectors. Much more research is clearly needed to understand the conditions and mechanisms that are responsible for the effects of adverse loading on bone.

Does the incidence of parafunction correlate with the incidence of implant failures? If the answer were yes, it would have been easy to argue for the relevance of the occlusal adverse load theory. However, this correlation (although often suspected) has never been confirmed in rigorous research. Many accounts have been published citing parafunctional behaviors as the source of implant failure. Yet, the incidence of parafunctional behavior in the general population exceeds by several fold the incidence of implant failure. Blaming every failure of a loaded implant on parafunction or adverse load seems more of a convenient excuse than a legitimate explanation. Thus, while parafunctional behaviors undoubtedly influence the incidence of mechanical complications (such as loosening of prosthetic components, accelerated wear, or fracture), the connection between biologic implant failures and parafunction is far more tenuous. Nonetheless, the following conclusions seem justified:

1. Differently induced interfacial micromotions may contribute to adverse cellular changes in the induction and maintenance of osseointegration.
2. In a manner that is similar to other healing responses, the quality of the developing or developed osseointegration response may vary. This time-dependent variability is influenced by general and local tissue health, the surgical protocol, and the subsequent loading.
3. The clinical relevance of such perceptions is that the clinician should employ optimal surgical technique and skill and seek to provide the best control possible of all forces acting on implants. This objective applies throughout both the initial healing and subsequent functional loading of the induced osseointegration response.

Overall, it is unknown why in some individuals the degree of osseointegration is great enough to cause mechanical failure from occlusal forces to occur at the level of the implant, implant framework, or component, while in other individuals the same occlusal forces leave the prosthetics intact and translate into a biologic failure at the bone-implant interface.

## The compromised healing/adaptation theory

Many years have been spent debating which of the two previous theories gives a more accurate account of osseointegration failure. This continuing controversy suggests that it is reasonable, indeed necessary, to look at alternative possibilities. Therefore, a third theory—compromised healing/adaptation—is proposed. This theory seeks to reconcile the differences in circumstances surrounding implant failure and to provide a framework on which to consider all types of failure. They include those that would be considered early (unloaded and noninfectious) failures and those that occur after loading or after the time-dependent insult of plaque-induced mucositis has altered the peri-implant environment.

The human jawbones manifest locally and systemically influenced characteristics that can profoundly influence whether the desired prerequisite of interfacial osteogenesis will take place. Just as important, some of these same factors as well as additional ones will influence whether osseointegration will be maintained once the implants are subjected to the demands of supporting a prosthesis that addresses the patient-mediated requirements of comfort, function, and esthetics. Ultimately, the clinician must consider whether the integrity of the host-implant interface is sufficient to endure the challenges placed on it in both the short and long term.

### Preloading failures

This chapter has alluded to compromised healing as a cause of implant failure. Compromised healing may occur as a result of some biologic malfunction or delay or as a result of harshness of a surgical intervention. It may very well be that the keys to implant success are the quality of bone healing and the strength of the osseointegration phenomenon. The quality of initial osseointegration is largely dependent on:

- Host factors that impact healing
- The quality of surrounding bone
- The quality of the surgical technique

Host factors (such as genetic predisposition, metabolic diseases, or nutritional status) affect healing, the incidence of infections, and the ability to deal with their consequences. The most common disease that impairs healing and is of relevance in the dental context is diabetes. Poorly controlled diabetes is a well-established risk for hindering successful osseointegration. In addition, as mentioned previously in this chapter, smoking increases the risk of implant failure, and evidence is beginning to mount that smoking increases early postloading failures; that is, implants in smokers are less able to withstand early functional demands. Those implants that do have sufficient osseointegration in the first year of function, regardless of smoking status, are likely to enjoy this sufficiency in the long run.

Bone quality (especially irradiated bone or poor type 4 bone found in the posterior maxilla or mandible) is intimately tied to the incidence of implant failure. The relevance of surgical skill and experience to success of surgical outcome is intuitive. For example, the failure rate for well-established surgeons who placed more than 50 implants was shown to be half the failure rate of less experienced surgeons who placed fewer than 50 implants.

Probably the single most important surgical determinant of implant success is ensuring that atraumatic bone preparation does not overheat the bone. Bone subjected to 47°C will become necrotic and, in this context, lose the implant. However, if the bone was overheated enough to damage the bone but not enough to lead to immediate implant failure, the implant will osseointegrate and survive and will appear to be just like every other implant. It is only after such an implant is subjected to loading that the lack of strength of the osseointegration response will become apparent. Because each implant is individually prepared with surgical drills, it is not surprising that within the same patient we may see a variable postsurgical response following placement of several implants—one implant site may be completely "burned" (and result in immediate implant loss), one site may be partially damaged (and result in late implant loss), and one site may be optimally prepared (and result in optimal osseointegration).

Slight bone necrosis always occurs after implant surgery. However, this is on a minimal scale, and the host cells are able to remove the necrotic debris successfully. When, on the other hand, the amount of necrotic debris overwhelms the body's defense mechanisms, a frank infection or an exudate-associated inflammatory response may result, giving the appearance of an infectious failure.

### Early postloading failures

*Early postloading implant failures* are made up of those that fail within the first 6 months of functional loading. The most likely cause is that, although the implants appeared clinically immobile during prosthesis fabrication, once subjected to functional forces, the interface could not withstand the forces applied to it. In these instances, it is likely that the radiographic appearance and apparent clinical immobility hid the fact that the strength of the implant-bone interface was compromised. The cumulative effect of the challenges to this interface in the form of functional loading, plaque-induced inflammation, and/or compromised ability to respond to the challenges (such as poor host response secondary to diabetes or smoking) results in an interface that degenerates to the point that it overwhelms the implant-host system and becomes symptomatic (secondary infection, pain, and/or implant mobility).

Although the precise cause of failure in implants that fail in this 6-month postloading window can be debated, in our opinion, failure so soon after loading is strongly indicative of a compromised healing response and one that produced an interface that was unable to adapt to the functional challenges placed on it. Given that there are no clearly validated measures to define a successfully osseointegrated implant, this classification is useful and pragmatic because it permits clinicians to discuss expectations of success and failure in patient-oriented terms with an avenue for managing those expectations relative to the presenting conditions.

## Late postloading failures

*Late postloading failures* are those that occur after 6 months of loading. In this scenario, an initially sturdy host-implant interface may become compromised and regress to the point at which it can no longer withstand the functional demands placed on it. In essence, just as for early postloading failures, the host is unable to adapt to the challenges placed on the implant interface, and osseointegration is compromised. However, the timing pattern of implant failures over time strongly suggests that late postloading failures are less common than preloading or early postloading failures. This is especially true of commercially pure screw-type titanium implants with a machined surface placed ad modum Brånemark, for which there is a reasonable body of long-term evidence. Such a timing pattern also reassures that, once an implant attains a state of adaptation or osseosufficiency, the prognosis for its maintenance is good. This, of course, presents a greater emphasis yet on an understanding of patient factors and use of surgical skill to achieve osseointegration.

Nevertheless, some implants do fail after 6 months of loading. In this group, the same aforementioned concepts of bacterially induced infection and/or occlusal adverse loading are widely touted as the harbingers of doom. Indeed, it is the late postloading failure group that necessitates a greater appreciation for the compromised healing/adaptation theory. To seek one or two factors as the cause of implant failure is detrimental to treatment planning and clinical management success, especially because undue adherence to either or both concepts undermines an understanding of the factors needed to establish and maintain osseointegration.

It is imperative that all possible factors that could influence the host-implant interface be viewed through a filter that asks the question "How will this factor influence the ability of the host, especially the response of osseous tissues, to adapt to functional demands?" When each factor is viewed separately, it is clear that most host-implant interfaces do establish with sufficiency and predictability. However, at specific times when the host response is compromised or a synergy from a multitude of factors results, the net effect is to confront the host's ability to adapt to the challenge with more than it can handle. Ultimately, the clinician must always respect the tolerance of the host-implant interface and never assume that it can meet all of the challenges. Rather, he or she must strive, through judicious treatment planning and prosthesis fabrication, to ensure that the adaptability threshold of the interface is never seriously tested.

The suboptimal adaptation theory is not an explanatory panacea. It, too, carries certain disadvantages. For example, to this day, despite numerous attempts to measure the quality of osseointegration—torque at placement, Periotest (Gulden), resonance frequency analysis—the predictive value of these measures is limited at best. Unfortunately, there are no accurate measures that would unequivocally establish the quality of osseointegration of a given implant and therefore enable the clinician to make an appropriate treatment decision. There is no way of establishing the adaptability of an individual's host-implant interface or if the bone was actually damaged in some way during the surgery.

## CONCLUSION

Three theories have been described to account for osseointegration failure: infection, adverse load, and compromised healing/adaptation. All three have degrees of merit and proponents and opponents. The infection theory arose from the periodontal literature and sought to draw analogies between the pathogenesis of periodontal disease and the pathogenesis of implant failure. This theory is supported by occasional observation of signs of inflammation and infection that precede, accompany, or follow loss of osseointegration and subsequent resolution of the inflammatory process with removal of the implant. This theory has difficulty accounting for implant failure in completely edentulous patients or in patients with impeccable oral hygiene and is largely incompatible with the known epidemiology of implant failure over time.

The adverse load theory, on the other hand, draws its inspiration from basic engineering principles. It is supported by a suspected correlation between the incidence of repeated prosthetic component failure and failure of implants. Yet it clearly cannot account for failure of implants prior to loading or for their failure under clearly minimal loading conditions. The authors prefer the theory of compromised healing/adaptation, which underscores the preeminence of the healing response in the induction of osseointegration.

The reader is encouraged to conclude that, as in everything else in life, there is no substitute for quality performance. Optimal healing will occur if basic surgical principles are meticulously followed and are combined with proper patient and site selection. Competent prosthodontic planning and restoration initiate and complete implant treatment.

Although there is no way to definitively test the quality of osseointegration, often common sense can be used as a good guide. The current fascination with immediate placement and immediate loading only makes sense if conditions are optimal. Premature enthusiasm under suboptimal conditions is likely to lead to another immediate event: immediate failure.

When host and site conditions are clearly not ideal (for example, when bone quality or quantity is very poor or there is a known history of implant failure), it is often advisable to follow these simple principles:

- *Wait.* Allow as much healing time postsurgically as possible.
- *Compensate.* Compensate for deficits in bone quality or quantity by modifying implant parameters under the clinician's control. Increase implant length, diameter, or number, while decreasing the length of cantilevers and narrowing the occlusal tables.
- *Do not overlook the merits of provisional prosthodontic treatment.* The ultimate test of any implant occurs only after it is loaded. Where there is any doubt about the quality of osseointegration (because of either surgical complications or radiographic evidence of significant bone loss in the first few months after placement), it is best to manage the situation with a provisional restoration before the clinician and the patient commit to the expense and the time needed to fabricate the definitive restoration. The premise is similar to the one adopted for demanding esthetic situations: design, wait, and reevaluate before a definitive design is prescribed. Loss of a loaded implant under a provisional restoration is still an unfortunate event, but one that carries a diminished fiscal outcome. A well-made laboratory-fabricated provisional restoration can last for years, yet at a fraction of the cost of the definitive restoration. Following a period of successful loading (ie, 1 to 2 years—the time span following loading when the vast majority of implant failures occur), the fabrication of a definitive restoration can then proceed.

This chapter provides only a brief summary of a very complex, fascinating, and incompletely understood topic. Nonetheless, it seeks a broad appreciation for a better understanding of the healing phenomenon as an integral part of the osseointegration technique.

## ACKNOWLEDGMENT

The authors wish to acknowledge Dr Kirk Preston for his contribution to "The occlusal adverse load theory" section of this chapter.

## RECOMMENDED READING

deLuca S, Zarb G. The effect of smoking on osseointegrated dental implants. 2. Peri-implant bone loss. Int J Prosthodont 2006;19:560–566.

Duyck J, Ronold HJ, Van Oosterwyck H, Naert I, Vander Sloten J, Ellingsen JE. The influence of static and dynamic loading on marginal bone reactions around osseointegrated implants: An animal experimental study. Clin Oral Implants Res 2001;12:207–218.

Esposito M, Hirsch J-M, Lekholm U, Thomsen P. Biological factors contributing to failures of osseointegrated oral implants. 1. Eur J Oral Sci 1998;106:527–551.

Esposito M, Hirsch J-M, Lekholm U, Thomsen P. Biological factors contributing to failures of osseointegrated oral implants. 2. Eur J Oral Sci 1998;106:721–764.

Frost HM. A 2003 update of bone physiology and Wolff's Law for clinicians. Angle Orthod 2004;74:3–15.

Geng JP, Tan KBC, Liu GR. Application of finite element analysis in implant dentistry: A review of the literature. J Prosthet Dent 2001;85:585–598.

Isidor F. Influence of forces on peri-implant bone. Clin Oral Implants Res 2006;17(suppl 2):8–18.

Lambert PM, Morris HF, Ochi S. Positive effect of surgical experience with implants on second-stage implant survival. J Oral Maxillofac Surg 1997;55(suppl 5):12–18.

Lindquist LW, Carlsson GE, Jemt T. A prospective 15-year follow up study of mandibular fixed prostheses supported by osseointegrated implants. Clinical results and marginal bone loss. Clin Oral Implants Res 1996;7:329–336.

Nevins M, Langer B. The successful use of osseointegrated implants in the treatment of the recalcitrant periodontal patient. J Periodontol 1995;66:150–157.

Quirynen M, De Soete M, van Steenberghe D. Infectious risks for oral implants: A review of the literature. Clin Oral Implants Res 2002;13:1–19.

Quirynen M, Peeters W, Naert I, Coucke W, van Steenberghe D. Peri-implant health around screw-shaped c.p. titanium machined implants in partially edentulous patients with or without on-going periodontitis. Clin Oral Implants Res 2001;12:589–594.

Sbordone L, Barone A, Ciaglia RN, Ramaglia L, Iacono VJ. Longitudinal study of dental implants in a periodontally compromised population. J Periodontol 1999;70:1322–1329.

Stanford CM, Brand RA. Toward an understanding of implant occlusion and strain adaptive bone modeling and remodeling. J Prosthet Dent 1999;81:553–561.

# 12

# STANDARDS OF CARE

KIRK PRESTON

The medical community has for many years embraced the concept of standard of care, which has resulted in numerous clinical guidelines for its practitioners. Terms such as *standard of care*, *evidenced-based practice*, and *clinical practice guidelines* became medical literature buzzwords and have now become popular and recurrent themes in dentistry. This is very much the case in the area of dental implant therapy, as peer-reviewed dental journals and other publications seek to provide guidelines for dentists about how to best provide the optimal standard of care for patients.

## DEFINITIONS OF STANDARD OF CARE

Although practitioners would agree that they must ethically provide the best care for their patients, the objective of standard of care remains imperfectly defined from both the legal and clinical perspectives. Definitions for *standard of care* include: "the *process* that a clinician should follow in a particular case," "the level at which the average, prudent provider in a given community would practice," and "how similarly qualified practitioners would manage the patient's care under the same or similar circumstances."[1] There are also other possible descriptions of standard of care; it could mean whatever expert witnesses determine it to mean or be interpreted as whatever therapy would have resulted in the best clinical outcome. A commonly accepted, clinically embedded definition is "whatever a majority of dentists would have done if faced with the same situation."

Legal and clinical impressions of what is meant by standard of care have their shortcomings. Standards of care developed by experts can be biased and can contain subjective elements. Accepting the principle of "the majority rules" as the definition of standard of care is not always acceptable either. Some would argue that advances in dentistry and medicine are not always supported by the majority and that, in medicine at least, some advances have spent years in the obscurity of minority opinion.

Still others have argued that the most valuable definition of standard of care is derived when an unbiased expert witness defines it by reference to evidence-based literature. Thus, it is apparent that what is meant by standard of care is complex and poorly understood by both clinical practitioners and the legal community. In short, a universally accepted, pragmatic working definition of standard of care is lacking in medicine and dentistry.

While strict definitions for what is meant by standard of care may never be universally accepted by the dental and legal communities, the criteria for a successful conceptual framework, or a working definition, might be more readily agreed on. Most practitioners would agree that the standard of care must reflect the complex and evolutionary nature of dentistry and the variability of acceptable ways to approach given patient or clinical situations. For example, there are numerous potential therapeutic interventions available to manage edentulism. These include complete dentures, implant-supported removable overdentures with various designs, and implant-supported fixed prosthetic solutions. Obviously, many of these technical solutions were not available many years ago, so it is important that the definition of standard of care reflect the temporal aspect of improved clinical therapeutic interventions. To complicate matters, despite many modern solutions to old dental problems such as edentulism, different contingents of practitioners, even within the same specialty, will endorse different but acceptable therapeutic solutions and offer differing opinions as to what is the best treatment.

Another desirable criterion for a definition of standard of care is clarity so that it is understandable to the practitioner. Most clinicians likely possess a limited understanding of what standard of care means and are unfamiliar with its specific definition. Nevertheless, it is not acceptable as a legal defense, either in a negligence lawsuit or in a proceeding by a government regulator on professional misconduct, for a practitioner to say that he or she was unaware of or did not understand the standard of care.

To summarize, the definitions and statements of standard of care should reflect ever-changing therapeutic approaches, recognize multiple approaches to dealing with clinical situations, and be easily understood by the average practitioner. In the context of these criteria, it is relevant to examine a recently published, popularly accepted statement on the management of the edentulous mandible. The *McGill Consensus Statement on Overdentures* states that "[t]he evidence currently available suggests that the restoration of the edentulous mandible with a conventional denture is no longer the most appropriate first choice prosthetic treatment. There is now overwhelming evidence that a 2-implant overdenture should become the first choice of treatment for the edentulous mandible."[2] Indeed, while this relatively new technique is certainly an acceptable approach in certain clinical situations, the statement falls short of acceptable criteria for standard of care in that it fails to recognize multiple approaches to dealing with similar clinical situations.

It must be remembered that the technique is a simple and logical extension of the report by Adell et al, who introduced a new paradigm for managing edentulism. It was followed by the Toronto Replication Study, wherein the treated edentulous population was made up exclusively of "prosthodontically maladaptive" patients. Both the 1991 and follow-up publications underscored the merits of the technique from both an efficacy and effectiveness standpoint. They also made a compelling case for a common need to achieve a stable prosthesis if prosthodontic adaptation is to occur. Therefore, it is tempting to conclude that all edentulous patients would benefit from the enhanced prosthesis security inherent in implant prosthodontics.

This also suggests that the McGill consensus reported a self-evident outcome while failing to differentiate real patient prosthodontic needs. This may also suggest a cynical interpretation that a commodity approach was inadvertently endorsed: If an item or technique is useful for special needs, it might as well be promoted universally, irrespective of whether it is needed or not.

The consensus statement also failed to acknowledge that adverse changes in the opposing arch might develop on a time-dependent basis, given the implicit changes in force concentration on maxillary denture-supporting tissues. There may also be a temporal element to this new treatment modality, and future research may lead to the emergence of even newer treatment options. It would appear that the McGill statement falls more in line with clinical practice guidelines than it does with a universally accepted standard of care.

# DEVELOPMENT OF CLINICAL PRACTICE GUIDELINES

The terms *clinical practice guidelines*, referring to plans designed mainly to guide the practitioner in dealing with clinical problems, and *standard of care*, which has its origin in the medicolegal community, are often used interchangeably. However, there are differences between these two terms. Clinical practice guidelines offer the practitioner particular, and often very specific, approaches to dealing with clinical situations and ideally should be based on the best available evidence in the literature. For example, in treating an otherwise healthy young patient with congenitally missing maxillary lateral incisors whose adjacent teeth are healthy, a reasonable clinical guideline would be to place dental implant-supported prostheses in that area. There are, of course, many clinical scenarios for which clinical practice guidelines have been developed. When such a treatment recommendation is compared against the criteria of what is meant by standard of care, such a recommendation falls short on acknowledging that treatment options may change with time, and it virtually eliminates other clinically acceptable treatment modalities.

Clinical practice guidelines relate to standard of care in that they are meant to provide the best possible care for the patient, if the practitioner adheres to certain clinical procedures. On the other hand, standard of care may be viewed as a reflection of the many complex components that are required for acceptable management of the patient's care in the eyes of the dental and legal communities. For example, in the aforementioned clinical scenario, it is not known whether the potentially negative outcomes of implant therapy were explained to the patient and whether the advantages and disadvantages of other treatment options were discussed. Clinical practice guidelines, with their narrow focus and potential time-dependent limitations, should not be construed as a substitute for standard of care, but should rather be seen as an element within the standard of care paradigm.

Clinical practice guidelines originate from a variety of sources, including product manufacturers, advocacy groups such as dental associations, and regulatory agencies, such as the Quality Assurance Committee of the Royal College of Dentists of Ontario, which have a mandate to provide guidelines to the profession. In Canada, the guidelines developed by regulatory bodies are in keeping with the legislation of the Dentistry Act and the Regulated Health Professions Act, and, from a legal perspective, have a higher level of authority than those issued from advocacy groups or product manufacturers.

In the absence of an alternative method of linking quality clinical care to the findings of evidence-based research and commonsense empirical approaches, practice guidelines do have their place, albeit with inherent shortcomings, and should be used cautiously. Attempts to adapt a universal therapeutic approach, often espoused in advertising from dental implant manufacturers for patients with missing teeth, fail to acknowledge that patients present with uniquely challenging clinical and biologic variations of edentulism. For example, the edentulous patient with morphologically challenging supporting structures could undergo a very complex surgical and prosthetic rehabilitation should an implant-supported prosthetic approach be recommended. In certain situations, finances or patient expectations might make traditional approaches such as conventional dentures more successful choices for therapeutic intervention.

Practitioners must accept that there are multiple acceptable ways to treat given patients or clinical scenarios and learn to question the purported high external validity (from implant manufacturers) of applying similar implant-supported treatments to the majority of patients in their practice. As previously discussed, clinical practice guidelines often fail to recognize that there are different therapeutic solutions that are acceptable to a significant contingent of practitioners, even from within the same specialty. There are, of course, practical limitations to clinical guidelines, such as how the guidelines are to be disseminated to the average practitioner, who will pay for the development and long-term administration of the guidelines, and how the clinician will manage potentially conflicting guidelines from different organizations and manufacturers. Clinical practice guidelines, when their limitations are understood, can be a useful adjunct for the practitioner who is developing treatment plans in the context of providing the best standard of care for patients.

# DEVELOPMENT OF A STANDARD OF CARE

Assuming that the criteria for standard of care can be agreed on, it is necessary to design a reasonable *process* for the development of a standard of care statement that is applicable for particular clinical situations. The two most common approaches are the *expert opinion method* and the *survey method*, both of which have advantages and disadvantages. The expert opinion method is self-explanatory and is often used in the legal community. The survey method, which is increasingly popular and is also used within the legal community, surveys a peer group of dentists to obtain input on customary and reasonable standards of practice.

The advantage of using the expert opinion model for developing standard of care statements is that it is a traditional method that is widely accepted. One disadvantage of this approach is that a distorted picture of standard of care might arise out of practice differences between general dentists and specialists. This problem is again reflected in reported standard of care guidelines for management of edentulous mandibles. The McGill consensus statement was developed by a panel of experts and specialists who, for the most part, were prosthodontists, and it appears to have been popularly accepted. However, such a therapeutic approach using dental implant–supported prostheses to manage edentulous mandibles is perhaps different from the approach used by the mainstream general dentist. Unfortunately, these opinions can be skewed by the biases that effect human judgment.

Consider the hypothetical scenario of the dentist who chose to not treat edentulous patients, or to not "do pink." This practitioner may now feel confident that the relatively easy availability of a simple surgical protocol that yields two to three abutments would not require the same technical demands for fabricating a mandibular complete denture. Hence it is time to recruit edentulous patients into the practice. What may be overlooked by the clinician is that implants are an adjunct to oftentimes very challenging complete-denture fabrication and not a tidy and simple little panacea.

Another concern in using the expert opinion approach as the basis for establishing standard of care statements is that expert opinion ranks very low on the hierarchical level of evidence as espoused by evidence-based practice guidelines, and there is the potential for this questionable approach to masquerade as evidence-based dentistry. On the other hand, randomized controlled trials are in short supply for various treatment modalities in dentistry in general, and implant dentistry specifically. Given the dearth of quality research, there is often little choice but to rely on either individual expert opinion or expert opinions from special interest groups.

The advantage of using a survey system is that it may help neutralize the effect of special interest groups, such as particular dental specialists, and provide more objective and accurate information about the standard of care. The question of which process would be most appropriate for use in the development of standard of care statements as they apply to dentistry must be addressed by the dental community.

# BIOETHICAL CONSIDERATIONS

Apart from the aforementioned limitations, the largely unexplored relationship between bioethics and clinical guidelines raises concerns about possible moral and ethical imperatives of clinical guidelines. Development or modification of clinical guidelines for the purpose of advocacy is grossly unethical and has potential negative repercussions for patients and the profession alike. A clinical example of this is the approach, advocated by a dental implant manufacturer, for managing edentulous patients with severe bone loss in the posterior mandible. The manufacturer recommends using a so-called all-on-four concept as a technique to avoid bone grafting, although there are presently very few long-term studies to support this surgical approach. In such situations it may be unethical for the manufacturers to advocate this approach without solid clinical data to support its success, and for the same reasons it might be equally unethical for clinicians to adopt this technique. The clinician should be cognizant of differences in reported treatment outcomes between manufacturers of dental implants and unbiased academic institutions.

The topic of industry- or manufacturer-supported or -initiated research is brilliantly reviewed in a provocative, must-read article by Lewis et al. The article addressed the risk of industry-supported university research as an incentive to promote the positive and suppress the negative. It went on to quote Francis Bacon's observation that "the human intellect…is more moved and excited by affirmatives than negatives." The paper concludes that "some bargains are Faustian and some horses are Trojan," with the advice that all of us who do research that is commercially supported should "dance carefully with the porcupine" and know in advance the price of intimacy.[3]

An ethical dilemma for the practitioner can arise when the clinical practice guidelines, often referred to as *standard of care guidelines* and sometimes developed by special interest groups, are not followed by the practitioner, yet a reasonable level of care outside the guidelines was delivered. In other words, in situations where there is a deviation from the clinical guidelines, is treatment considered unethical per se, and would it be unethical to evaluate new treatments that represent a significant departure from the currently accepted standard of care? In the case of the previously discussed edentulous patient, if the dentist had placed a traditional, economically affordable prosthesis as opposed to an implant-supported prosthesis, would the patient have been shortchanged? Was the dentist acting ethically and in good faith? It might even be possible for some guidelines to be so specific that they expose practitioners to liability when their actions fall outside of rigid protocols. It is evident that there are many ethical and moral implications of stating standard of care guidelines.

Morally and ethically, clinicians owe it to their patients to maintain an adequate standard of care during treatment. Critics of clinical guidelines have also suggested that guidelines undermine the dentist's autonomy and minimize the exercise of professional judgment, thereby potentially compromising the patient's standard of care. In the previous example where the use of implant-supported overdentures for edentulous patients was advocated as the standard of care, some critics would argue that these statements, which are tantamount to clinical practice guidelines, remove clinical decision making from the practitioner and form the basis of collective policy making.

Many faithful proponents of evidence-based dentistry would support the view that only the results of well-designed randomized controlled trials should govern the standard of care relating to therapeutic interventions and form the basis for establishing clinical practice guidelines. When evidence from randomized controlled trials is lacking in a given area of dentistry, some might argue that there is no acceptable standard of care and that practitioners are acting in an ethical void. Most would agree that there is at least a trend that standards of care are increasingly defined by the best available evidence rather than by local practice standards or the often idiosyncratic opinions of experts. Given the current accessibility of literature, it is perhaps the responsibility of the clinician to keep up with the latest evidence, and to practice without doing so may be considered unethical.

The challenge facing those who develop guidelines is to determine how these ethical issues might be addressed in the process of development and to reach moral consensus on the many bioethical issues involved. Pragmatically, they must determine how ethically sound guidelines that also reflect innovative and promising, but perhaps clinically unproven, therapeutic interventions can be developed.

Although there is no easy solution to this problem, the practitioner must be educated on how to critically evaluate current literature and know how to implement the findings in practice at the individual patient level. Setting individual clinical guidelines based on an analysis of the literature and within the context of the standard of care, as opposed to mass-produced clinical guidelines, is a reasonable first step toward addressing this problem. The major advantage of this approach is that, over time, personalized clinical guidelines can be removed, modified, and improved to better reflect the ever-changing advances in therapy. The ethical limitations of using new treatment approaches are minimized over time as the literature improves.

What, then, are the ethical implications for practitioners operating without some form of clinical guidelines? For many clinical situations, clinical guidelines may not apply, or even exist, because at present the volume of clinical guidelines, though increasing, is still small in relation to the scope of clinical care. The uniqueness of individual patient characteristics and the complex treatment planning in certain patients can also be at odds with treatment recommendations based on clinical guidelines, if they exist. There are many previously unencountered or very complicated situations to be addressed in the course of daily practice, especially when implants are used. Is the practitioner who must treat a situation with no clinical guidelines operating in an ethical void? Is the dentist who, with the best of intentions, simply "does things differently," mainly because there are no guidelines available, in serious ethical, and perhaps legal, jeopardy?

Failure to refer a patient to an appropriate specialist when complicated clinical situations beyond the expertise of the practitioner arise not only would be unethical but also would be an act of professional misconduct that would be seen in the civil courts as negligent. Unlike in medicine, where referrals to an appropriate specialist by the general practitioner are routine and often financially remunerated, in dentistry referrals to dental specialists are often cumbersome and financially punitive for the general practitioner. For example, in dentistry there is no recognized specialty in implantology; therefore, the general dentist has to decide whether to refer the patient to an oral surgeon, a periodontist, or a prosthodontist. Even with the best of intentions *to* refer, it is not always easy for the general dentist to decide *where* to refer. For example, for the routine procedure of maxillary sinus grafting, should the general dentist refer to the periodontist or the oral surgeon? Realistically, there is a lack of consensus within the specialist community with respect to these situations. The ethical challenge is for the general dentist to make the appropriate referral, and patients may be morally wronged if the referral was inappropriately directed.

In medicine and dentistry it is well accepted that it is unethical to undertake particular procedures without adequate training, and such action constitutes professional misconduct and negligence. Unfortunately there are no guidelines or regulations available, at least in Canada, as to what level of skill is required for the surgical and prosthetic rehabilitation of patients. Training is offered through many sources, including specialty programs in dental schools, private academic institutions often operated by specialists, implant company–sponsored events, and, more recently, at the undergraduate level at dental schools. However, as previously mentioned, there is no one specialty in this area, and the nature of what constitutes adequate training is left up to the practitioner. The ethical dilemma facing the practitioner is that adequate training is needed to apply appropriate therapy but that without experience it is difficult to choose the training that will enable him or her to manage the complexity of the case in question.

## ECONOMIC ANALYSIS

Economic analysis of new and established medical interventions has increasingly become the focus of research over the past two decades. Expensive clinical interventions, combined with limited health care budgets (at both societal and personal levels), demand a better deployment of resources and identification of relevant alternatives. While the economic analyses of dental implant–supported interventions are limited, the number of proposed standard of care statements has increased.

Clinical practice guidelines and economic analyses share similarities in that they both start with a particular patient population, a clinical problem, and a set of treatment alternatives. However, their outcomes in terms of what is considered best practice are usually quite different. An economic analysis examines the most efficient allocations of resources and tries to maximize the treatment outcome while minimizing the outlay of resources. Clinical practice guidelines are intended to guide the practitioner in providing the most effective outcomes and are not necessarily cost related. Consequently, proponents of economic guidelines for management of edentulous patients would be unlikely to offer dental implant therapy as a best practice because of its high costs, whereas professionally popular clinical practice guidelines recommend dental implant therapy as the most effective treatment for edentulous patients. This once again raises an ethical issue for the practitioner who must choose between a clinically effective, but potentially more expensive, therapy or a less effective and more affordable treatment.

The solution to this dilemma may be to integrate economic analysis and clinical practice guidelines. Given that economic considerations are often a major limiting factor in patient acceptance of prosthodontic treatment and that new technologies and their application increase total treatment costs, an argument can be made for incorporating an economic analysis into clinical practice guidelines. For example, current implant therapy is inarguably efficacious and effective for specific clinical situations. Yet, more rigorous long-term outcome results about predictability and cost-effectiveness are required before an across-the-board, implants-only clinical strategy should be considered.

The oral rehabilitation of edentulous patients in particular should be a prime target for such economic analyses. Edentulism is, after all, a common problem in elderly people, whose limited physical and economic resources frequently preclude extensive and expensive treatment. It is apparent that a simple and effective treatment technique is required to accommodate their needs.

There is a dearth of information pertaining to the economic burden for patients seeking treatment with tissue-integrated prostheses. Available economic studies, mainly on edentulous patients, have considered clinical costs from the clinician's viewpoint and compared implant-supported prostheses with conventional complete dentures. Short-term studies have reported that implant-supported restorations are more expensive than conventional dentures. However, longer-term studies that also included analyses of maintenance costs suggested that the cost difference between implant-supported and conventional prostheses may not be all that dissimilar. Long-term studies have also observed that the overdenture retained with a resilient bar retention mechanism is more cost-effective than the fixed prosthesis for rehabilitation of the edentulous mandible. Patient satisfaction and oral health–related quality of life improved significantly if a mandibular denture was implant supported.

In addition, these studies have addressed the issue of maintenance, which should be discussed with patients so that they may reach scientifically based decisions. It is important that patients understand the implications of treatment and appreciate that costs will be accrued in the future for maintenance purposes. Unfortunately, economic studies comparing different prosthetic techniques in partially edentulous patients are extremely limited, precluding any conclusions.

If the argument for the incorporation of economic analysis into clinical practice guidelines is accepted, there are some potential problems in reconciling the two camps. One of the challenges is finding acceptable, agreed on economic outcomes for the developers of clinical practice guidelines. Indeed, the measurement of outcomes is problematic, because different members of society may have different opinions on the relevance of outcome measurements. A variety of indicators, such as Oral Health–Related Quality of Life and Quality-Adjusted Life Years, are available; however, there is no universal agreement or industry standard as to which is best to use.

Another potential problem in the development of clinical guidelines is the source of funding. To date, much of the clinical research in this area is supported directly or indirectly by profitable implant manufacturing companies, whereas economic analyses are most likely supported in university settings, with a more controlled bias. The different agendas may have to be reconciled prior to the development of clinical practice guidelines that include a component of economic analysis.

## CONCLUSION

New dental implant–based therapy is increasingly prescribed and researched as a routine alternative to traditional prosthodontic treatments. This approach is clearly a significant bio-

technologic advance, but it has elicited many unanswered and fundamentally broader questions relating to standard of care, clinical practice guidelines, bioethics, and economic analysis.

This chapter attempts to provide the reader with insights into the different concepts of standard of care and clinical practice guidelines. The dental community must reach a consensus about the specific relevance and meaning of these concepts in the context of the demands of evidence-based dentistry. The notion of routine practice of implant-based therapy in prosthodontics has also been challenged by the discussion of bioethical concerns, which must be more formally addressed through additional research. Finally, the importance of incorporating economic analysis into the development of clinical practice guidelines has been underscored.

## ACKNOWLEDGMENTS

The author wishes to acknowledge Dr Nikolai Attard for his contribution to the "Development of Clinical Practice Guidelines" and "Economic Analysis" sections of this chapter.

## REFERENCES

1. Banja JD. Ethics, case management, and the standard of care. Case Manager 2006;17:20–22.
2. Feine J. The McGill Consensus Statement on Overdentures: Mandibular two-implant overdentures as first choice standard of care for edentulous patients. Gerodontology 2002;19:3–4.
3. Lewis S, Baird P, Evans RG, et al. Dancing with the porcupine: Rules for governing the university-industry relationship. CMAJ 2001;165:783–785.

## RECOMMENDED READING

Adell R, Lekholm U, Rockler B, Brånemark P-I. A 15-year study of osseointegrated implants in the treatment of the edentulous jaw. Int J Oral Surg 1981;10:387–416.

Drummond MF, O'Brien B, Stoddard GL, Torrance GW. Methods for the Economic Evaluation of Health Care Programmes, ed 2. Oxford, England: Oxford University Press, 1997.

Empey M, Carpenter C, Jain P. Resident's perspective: What constitutes standard of care? Ann Emerg Med 2004;44:527–531.

Jones JW, McCullough LB, Richman BW. Standard of care: What does it really mean? J Vasc Surg 2004;40:1255–1257.

# FUTURE DIRECTIONS

CLARK STANFORD

Tooth replacement strategies have a long history in the culture of innovations that in time can lead to sufficient patient satisfaction. In the past, the choices made in these developments have often been clinician driven, and the assessment of the outcomes of care has been made with little input from the patient's perspective. This professional myopia is the greatest danger as the future unfolds. What the clinician chooses to see is what he or she will see. In today's electronic environment, the resources clinicians consult are the same as those that patients can and often do. Thus, dental professionals must be prepared to address, consult, defend, or refute positions that informed patients bring to the conversation. The ability of a white coat to deflect questions from patients or their legal advisers is long gone.

This view of the future is intended to lay a context for a vision of the future that covers, from the smallest of dimensions, the so-called nanoscale interactions, to the largest of daily interactions, the social implication of treatment. Innovations are occurring simultaneously at all of these levels. The clinician's knowledge will become obsolete, and it is his or her responsibility to recognize this fact and thus to stay current through the process of ongoing education. Innovations in the field of implant dentistry will range from improvements in bone and mucosal attachment and adhesion technologies to evolutions in governmental payment strategies. Are today's dental professionals ready?

## TECHNOLOGY

In its current form, a dental implant represents only one form of tooth replacement. The technology arose from one in which the surface did not elicit a reaction (either negative or positive). The future holds that implant surfaces will be capable as a platform to initially elicit a biologic response; to prevent, reduce, or manage such a response once it is underway; or to act as a drug delivery system.

One of the key areas for innovation is the increasing understanding of nanoscience. Although it appears to be the latest trendy term bandied about, it does have validity because the world behaves very differently at the nanolevel. The prefix *nano-* refers to structures or features on the order of 1 to 100 nm in dimension (a human hair, by contrast, is about 10,000 nm in diameter). Nanostructured materials behave in unique ways because of electrical, mechanical, physical, and biologic properties that are elevated in part by the increased degrees of surface that is exposed to interact with biologic molecules (also known as a *catalytic platform*).

In a series of studies used to determine the biologic influences of implant surfaces, an "optimal" 60-nm grain size ($\pm$10 nm) was shown to elicit an increase in cellular attachment, proliferation, and differentiation of osteoblasts. Cells were observed to attach preferentially to grain boundary regions, suggesting that in the presence of smaller grains (and thus more grain boundaries per surface area) there was more reactive area for bone healing. Molecular modeling has suggested that bone-forming cells (osteoblasts) bind at these sites, and the acquired cell shape appears to play a role in eliciting a bone-like differentiation phenotype.

One currently marketed implant surface (OsseoSpeed, Astra Tech) uses a titanium oxide–blasted and mildly etched surface to produce 60- to 100-nm surface pitting, allowing eventual secondary osseointegration (the end process of turnover of bone at the implant surface after a period of healing) on the macroscopic blasted surface, which allows for primary osseo-integration (stability). This surface has been shown to have osteoinductive behavior when modeled with human stem cells in vitro and to express specific bone-associated proteins in laboratory, animal, and human studies.

Laboratory and clinical research also has been published to support the outcomes of a titanium hydrophilic surface prepared by large-grit blasting and acid etching (SLActive, Straumann). Other manufacturers have used thin solution-based coatings of calcium and phosphate (eg, NanoTite, BIOMET/3i) or thin ion-spray amorphous (noncrystalline) calcium phosphate coatings (NanoTite Surface, Bicon). Unfortunately, there are few or no scientific studies on the latter two surfaces to support the putative claims of superiority over oxide-prepared commercially pure titanium surfaces. All of these technologies should be considered early developments in this area, because trials are currently underway with recombinant human bone morphogenetic protein 2 coatings on dental implants. Future developments in implant materials and surfaces will also be associated with short-term drug delivery systems and unique implant shapes and sizes.

Clinicians should be wary of quickly incorporating an implant system touted as "the latest and greatest" in their practice if:

- The new system is intended for a clinical procedure they are not comfortable with (eg, immediate provisionalization or self-drilling implant systems).
- Studies—either minimal laboratory or especially rigorous clinical research—have not been performed or are "ongoing."
- The system is provided by an unknown manufacturer (although this is not always the case).
- Marketing pressure by patients or colleagues appears to give a message that just seems too good to be true (which it normally is).

When all is said and done, clinicians must assess their own outcomes over time (eg, a minimum of 3 years) and determine if the implant systems they are using, with clinical procedures in which they have confidence, provide predictable results. The patient-level outcomes for the original turned-surface dental implant discussed earlier have a substantial level of predictabil-

ity that has not been clinically improved in the last 20 years, regardless of the claims of some manufacturers. Clinical mistakes are costly for the clinician but more costly for the patient.

The area of innovation in implant designs will probably occur in the area of the transmucosal abutment or transmucosal implant body design. For example, long-term outcomes with the external hex systems are now showing that 15 to 20 years following placement, an elevated level of implant perimucositis or minor associated bone loss may occur. While the clinical relevance of these observations may be questionable, attempts to address such a contingency seem relevant. For example, there already are abutment designs that make use of consus abutment connections, which are designed to provide abutment-implant stability and minimize the abutment-implant gap. The premise here is that this change will result in minimal chronic inflammatory infiltrate in the peri-implant mucosa. Currently attention is also being paid to designs that narrow the transmucosal abutment to develop a larger volume of mucosal tissue. This so-called platform switching makes use of the biologic nature of epithelia to attach to biomaterials based on the available surface area (versus a linear dimension) in an effort to prevent inflammation, thinning mucosa, and recession. In the future there will be more innovations with nanotopography designed to enhance expression of basement membrane proteins (eg, laminins).

Promising technologies also suggest the development of an artificial "cementum" may be possible, conveying similar properties of bone stability and mucosal integration into the transmucosal portion of the implant. The future will also see the progressively increased use of ceramic-based materials, such as yttria–partially stabilized zirconia, for the transmucosal abutment.

In addition to the refinements in materials, improvements in computer-aided dentistry (design) and computer-aided machining will provide flexibility in rapid prototyped custom abutments and even custom implant shapes and configurations. In part, one driving force in this area will be clinicians faced with maintaining an increasing number of "legacy" implants, either manufactured and placed years before but now off the market or from unidentifiable systems.

## PROCEDURES

As more clinicians use implants in various modes of therapy, an increasing number of them will be exposed to so-called cutting-edge procedures that may or may not have sufficient clinical evidence to support them. One ongoing area of interest is in expedited clinical therapies advocated by a smaller set of clinicians (eg, immediate loading). There will clearly be an expanded role for technologies, although this must be balanced with the increased costs of care. This will be an issue for the profession, if technology, rather than the needs and desires of patients, is driving innovations. This increased emphasis on technology, which increases the cost of care, could make tooth replacement therapies all the more an exclusive realm of the well-to-do.

The future does hold promise that the use of augmentation procedures such as recombinant bone-inductive proteins will be made available at a clinically useful price that would allow osseous site development to be performed by the general dentist in a minimally invasive manner. Coupling of these types of inductive materials with self-assembling rigid scaffold structures provides the promise of local site development though a simple in-office procedure. All of these proposed applications will come with costs and benefits to the educational community. Dental school curricula are already addressing the critical need for evidence-based care, and these types of materials and clinical procedures will be very useful applications of these principles for the private clinician.

In addition to the educational change at the dental school and postgraduate level, there is a political aspect to these developments. Dental specialists who have conventionally considered themselves to be the owners and providers of exclusive services will find increased competition (general dentists versus prosthodontists for complex restorations; prosthodontists versus periodontists versus oral surgeons for site development and implant placement). These tensions can have a significant side benefit: an expanded number of providers and the potential for increased competition, which will tend to hold or drive down the costs of care. In the end, this has the potential to improve patient access and care for more than the top-earning 3% of the population.

# PATIENT-CENTERED CARE

In the future, patients will increasingly advocate for their own treatment decisions. Part of this process will be the expectation that individual patients will be assessed based on their known genetic risk factors and will be provided with individualized treatment plans that efficiently and economically address these risk factors. One example of this is the recent interest in the relationship between habitual smoking and periodontal disease progression and possible increased implant failure. Dentists in the future will be called on to assess and address the impact of genetic and systemic risk factors and make treatment decisions based on these diagnostic frameworks. This is not a "medical model" of health care but a "healthy model" of care. For example, patients who present to the office may be easily diagnosed in the next few years with a handheld saliva detection system capable of detecting polymorphisms in the interleukin 1 gene family and/or the interleukin 1 receptor family that puts that patient at increased risk for periodontal disease, bone loss, and implant loss, especially if he or she has habits such as smoking. These types of simple clinical tests will aid the clinician chairside in diagnosis, patient counseling, and interventional treatment planning.

Treatment planning in some cases may include the use of chemotherapeutics (eg, host modulation therapies using tetracycline-like drugs to block matrix metalloproteinase pathways, preventing bone loss in the first place). Depending on when the patient enters the office, it may be possible to prevent, inhibit, or reverse the destruction commonly thought to occur with periodontitis. Although that may seem futuristic, it is already possible to assess the microbial and immune system genes as well as identify and separate pathologic from commensal host cells, tissues, and organisms. With chairside microarray-based technologies, there is a potential that dentists of the future will never need to treat a patient for tooth loss with a titanium implant.

Diagnosing genetic conditions may seem out of the scope of practice for dentists, but consider this example. A recent group has designed a means to transfer the missing or defective protein that results in a genetic condition called *hypohidrotic ectodermal dysplasia*. In this condition, patients present with thin hair, minimal sweat glands, frontal bossing, periorbital melanotic pigmentation, multiple missing teeth, and atrophic ridges. Recent studies have indicated that greater incidences of implant loss and complications occur in this population, reinforcing the idea that implant therapy is probably a transitional technology. In a recent set of studies, a group in Switzerland and collaborators in the United States have demonstrated in two animal models that they could identify the defective protein leading to the syndrome phenotype, design a maternal protein transfer system (based on antibody conjugation technologies), and deliver the correct protein (ED-1) to the neonatal animal, providing a complete reversal of the phenotypic anomalies (including all the normal teeth) in one or two doses given around birth. The hope and empowerment this gives to patients and their families is enormous, and the findings underscore the need for clinicians to stay current with the rapid applications of genomics and proteinomics to clinical health care.

Another driving force in changes at the patient level will be the impact of the increasing number of elderly patients and the increasing percentage that will not accept tooth loss as a part of aging. The older patient may have treatment demands and expectations that tax the diagnostic and treatment capabilities of a busy practitioner. As procedures with high value but low time expenditure, such as bleaching, have become increasingly popular, patients' desires and expectations for tooth replacement therapies that are minimally invasive have grown. Electronic access to multiple sources of health information (both good and bad) is available to patients, clinicians, and third-party entities. This has changed and will continue to change the practice of health care.

At the society and public health policy levels, there are likely to be groundswells of change in the near future. There already has been a radical increase in the number of companies making implant products and devices. Some of these companies enter the market seeking mostly profit with minimal investment in product documentation and research. As observed in the dental laboratory industry, it is possible that low-cost dental implants will emerge, adding economic pressure to reduce fees, especially downward pressure on fees paid by third parties. Although this prospect is of concern, it is possible that third-party payers may begin to dictate a level of reimbursement based on price and thus dictate a certain "preferred panel" of covered lower-cost implant systems. This would be a logical outcome, if the profession does not demand that all companies rigorously document clinical outcomes of the systems they provide.

One way to consider addressing the combined impacts of access to care (smaller number of dentists with an expanding population), the increasing number of elderly patients, and changes in styles of dental practice (part-time, transitional practice versus a career, etc) is to embrace new models of clinical dental practice care delivery. Although new models of care delivery are controversial at the political, social, and economic levels, the crushing demand may drive certain changes. One example is to consider delivery of care by dentist-supervised ancillary dental support personnel (denturist, advanced dental nurse practitioners, or the development of a form of a dental "physician's assistant"). The dentist would act in the role of the master diagnostician and manage treatment planning but delegate, with supervision, the technical phases of care. Such a groundswell has already happened in medicine, and it may be the near future of dentistry.

## CONCLUSION

Patients go to their dental professional with a complex array of wants, needs, and desires. The ability to provide a predictable life-restoring service, such as dental implant therapy, is an enormous advancement for dentistry, an advancement that has really only been accepted in this generation. The work of health care pioneers in the osseointegration field, such as Brånemark, Schroeder, Zarb, and Albrektsson, has enabled clinicians to offer a form of tooth replacement therapy that is minimally invasive and rather predictable. This only occurred after insightful and rigorous clinical assessment of outcomes, which were completed before these findings were presented to the dental community. This is an enormous legacy and responsibility for the current and future generations of clinicians and dental educators. Dentists must continue to provide the best care for patients with an eye to preventing disease and to providing evidence-based therapy to provide relief from disease.

The clinician provides implant-based tooth replacement for the rest of the patient's life. In no other area of dentistry is a procedure performed with the implicit assumption that part of the procedure (the bone-anchored implant) will be there for the rest of that patient's life. Further, a binding relationship is created by the dentist between that patient and a third party (an implant manufacturer), who may or may not have the same commitment that clinicians do to the long-term health of the patient. At the end of the day, for the good of patients and the reputation of the profession, clinicians must demand reliability, stability, and predictability from manufacturers of tooth replacement systems.

## RECOMMENDED READING

Albrektsson T. Direct bone anchorage of dental implants. J Prosthet Dent 1983;50:255–261.
Thomas JB, Peppas NA. Nanotechnology and biomaterials. In: Gogotsi Y (ed). Nanomaterials Handbook. Boca Raton, FL: CRC, 2006.

# FROM REARVIEW VISTAS TO CURRENT LANDSCAPES

GEORGE A. ZARB

It is tempting to conclude this book by reiterating the virtues of the phenomenon of osseointegration. Its emergence as a versatile, routine clinical technique has been a long and exciting journey that has spawned numerous learned organizations and educational initiatives. Above all, it has catalyzed extensive research, which in turn invigorated traditional synergies between clinical disciplines and their basic science counterparts. This is all very laudatory, and both the profession and patients have been its beneficiaries. However, the intellectual ferment resulting from osseointegration and its clinical treatment appeal also has a downside. The dramatic popularization of implant treatment and extensive commercial sponsorship of research and education in the field may now risk subverting the public interest.

Given such a context, a number of related concerns require emphasis, as this chapter takes stock of the current clinical landscape of surgical, prosthodontic, and biomaterials synergies plus other collaborations in implant dentistry:

• The implant
• The healing response
• The esthetic issue
• The oral ecology
• The research challenge

## THE IMPLANT

Implants continue to be introduced as variations on a theme of the original commercially pure titanium cylindrical screw. Virtually all currently marketed implants, irrespective of their different degrees of scientific pedigree, offer subtle and some-times even profound design shifts that are supposed to maximize and optimize the induced interfacial healing response. Yet in spite of the extraordinary documented success of osseointegration, there is much that remains imperfectly understood about the induced biologic process and its long-term effectiveness.

One apparent and irrefutable fact is that the inherent robustness of a host's healing potential encourages an induction of interfacial osteogenesis irrespective of the operator; the host bone site; the patient's sex, age, race, or behavioral habits; or traditional ecologic intraoral concerns. This realization has expedited a treatment culture that seems readily responsive to commercial directives. The implant industry has to a great extent fallen prey to the notion that healing is entirely dependent on initial implant stability. This idea encourages the perception that the right thread pattern will conquer all concerns; in the process, the surgical principles of training, skills, and scrupulous tissue handling risk falling between the cracks.

This has been the starting point for the numerous current market variations that incorporate convergent themes of implant material, size, and macroscopic and microscopic features (Fig 14-1). The resultant and hopefully scientifically determined, biomechanical qualities of any final implant product are an integral and vital part of the successful outcome equation. However, the imaging and selection of the proposed bone site, together with surgical skill in manipulation of host tissues are the inarguable major determinants of long-term treatment success. Any quality implant per se is only as efficacious as the skill and judgment of the operator who is placing it.

The longevity of the biologic response is inadequately documented for several of the implant systems in common use. However, this has clearly not deterred the commercial race to acquire a substantial share of a rapidly growing worldwide market.

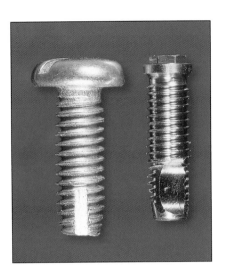

**Fig 14-1** The scientific trajectory from an ordinary screw *(left)* to a cylindrical, threaded implant design *(right)* is suggested by this image. It underscores macroscopic features that reconcile convenience of use with establishment of stability.

This reality makes for an exciting yet risky ongoing developmental climate. It certainly encourages interesting and entertaining presentations at meetings in the category of progress and new developments. A typical example is visual advertising of the evidence of maximum bone-to-implant contact as the yardstick of optimal clinical long-term outcomes. As a result, the race is on for the company with the highest bone-to-implant contact to claim to be the winner of the osseointegration stakes, even in the absence of outcome evidence.

The current enthusiasm for mini-implants and micro-implants is another obvious example. Historically, different-sized implants were used for a variety of reasons, such as avoidance of implant fractures and establishment of optimal ratios for bone support. The justification for employing such abbreviated implants is unclear, with evidence for their longevity far from compelling.

This current modus operandi does not always provide products that result from rigorous clinical testing. The rush to market implant components remains a far cry from the rigorous testing associated with the pharmacologic industry. This warning may sound didactic since a strong argument could also be advanced that progress from an established baseline of proven clinical efficacy, and to a large extent short-term effectiveness, cannot be expected to undergo the identical long-term scientific scrutiny demanded of the pioneering work of early clinical scientists. Nonetheless, the success of implants should continue to be measured by documented outcome evidence and not by sales results.

Yet, as discussed in chapter 13, ongoing research at a basic level remains full of promise. For example, it has already been shown that titanium implants with different surface topography modulate the expression of a specific set of genes that are not involved in osteotomy-induced wound healing. Moreover,

the induced gene products contribute to the establishment of osseointegration and may offer additional scope for an increased understanding of the mechanisms of osseointegration. Microroughened implant surfaces have also been shown to speed up the process of osseointegration. They are reported to have advantages over the original machined and relatively smooth surfaces by providing better mechanical interlock as well as promoting osteoblastic differentiation that results in faster bone formation. This well-supported observation quickly led to earlier implant-loading protocols, although the desired long-term outcomes and advantages of this approach's leap of faith remain far from compelling. In fact, the scientific jury is still out on the issue.

Furthermore, the current explosion of interest in nanotechnology for industrial and medical uses suggests enormous promise for yet another scientifically driven generation of implant designs. Nanotechnology-based surface modification processes may very well yield novel properties and functions and profoundly influence cellular behavior. The hoped-for outcome of such a development would then be the possibility of an enhanced ability to control osseointegration. Although an additional design leap to incorporating more microroughness on a nanoscale may seem logical and desirable in both orthopedics and dentistry, clinical prudence demands more scientific evidence to justify a declaration of a new generation of implants that can lead to even better osseointegration.

It is always tempting to get carried away by the aura of new scientific claims and believe that "success in a package" can be readily purchased. Although the quality of scientific evidence that characterizes a particular implant and its ongoing improvement can be assessed, even a well-established implant product remains only one side of the therapeutic coin. The clinician's judgment, skill, and integrity will always comprise the other side.

# THE HEALING RESPONSE

It has been repeatedly argued in this book that successful long-term osseointegration outcomes result from well-planned and scrupulous exploitation of bone's healing response. This clinical fact has now been robustly documented in patients from both sexes, different races, and across the age spectrum—a reflection of the extraordinary efficacy of the applied clinical technique. It has also proven to be successful in patients whose overall systemic health may be compromised but not in a brittle state, as well as in patients who have undergone the rigors of oncologic therapy. The bottom line is that virtually every host bone site is a legitimate candidate for implant placement. If the site fits into a proposed treatment plan that includes a preprosthetic surgical protocol, an implant-supported and -retained prosthesis becomes a compelling consideration.

While cognizant of these truisms, clinicians were initially frustrated whenever patients needing implant treatment lacked host site dimensions to accommodate implant placements. Several oral and maxillofacial surgeons sought to compensate for these restrictions by employing autogenous bone grafts. The approach was for a long time the gold standard in orthopedic surgery and similarly provided the selected osseointegration site with an osteoconductive matrix together with vital cellular and growth-stimulating features.

Many patients benefited from such ingenious and virtuoso surgical interventions, but the risk of attendant morbidity was always present, even in healthy patients. In fact, the disadvantages of limited host harvesting sites, increased postoperative pain, and risk of infection militated against the procedure's routine use. Moreover, patients with compromised health pictures also seemed to run an increased risk of ensuing morbidity, thereby limiting the protocol's application even further.

The promise of regenerative medicine dramatically changed the surgical approach to smaller, depleted potential host bone sites. Three-dimensional biomaterial scaffolds or matrices were introduced to support the regeneration of the lost tissues, and the method rapidly became a routine one, especially in smaller host sites. However, long-term clinical observation and a mixed quality of documentation underscored the fact that, while such passive therapeutic matrices proved useful in the provision of a framework and maintenance of a space for tissue deposition, unpredictable results (eg, soft tissue dehiscence) were not infrequent, and the size of the targeted site was a frequent treatment deterrent. Considerable debate has ensued in the literature and at scientific meetings. The efficacy of osseointegration and its dependence on prolonged barrier function—whether such membranes should be cross linked or not—continues to elicit serious debate and treatment challenges.

Even more recently, claims that endorse recombinant growth factor therapeutics have been promulgated. The suggestion is that vertical bone augmentation is no longer the exclusive domain of the onlay graft, with all of its unpredictability. As a result, sinus augmentation and alveolar ridge augmentation, with or without associated tooth extractions, are reported as being feasible and indeed desirable. A new sense of optimism in this next phase of the ongoing management of so-called site improvement was launched. Early evidence of postoperative de novo bone formation was rapidly translated into increased surgical application and of course sales for the companies whose products claim to "finally bring osteogenesis under the control of surgeons." All of this is heady and exciting stuff and clearly promising. Yet the question has to be repeatedly asked: Does the new technique demonstrate the same predictable and reproducible results that underscored the introduction of osseointegration in the first place? Clinical prudence continues to demand an ongoing commitment to robust evidence-based information before such promising claims are readily incorporated into routine clinical practice.

# THE ESTHETIC ISSUE

Both general dental practitioners and dental specialists are health care givers who undertake the professional responsibility of ensuring continuing oral health and function in an esthetically satisfactory oral milieu. The disciplines of orthodontics, maxillofacial surgery, and prosthodontics, in particular, regard such objectives as integral parts of their mandate. The roots of all three specialties remain inseparable from an overriding commitment to control and manage disease, traumatic and dyscrasia-related processes, and their sequelae.

However, in the consumer marketplace, the pursuit of "feeling better" is frequently measured in terms of self-esteem, leading to a blurring between cosmetic and dental health care. An esthetically pleasing natural or restored dentition is an integral and important part of the individual's self-image. In North America in particular, the middle class and the wealthy regard straight, white teeth as a virtual birthright. Yet the move into beautification tends to turn the patient into an object, an easel on which the dentist can seek to be creative. The present cosmeticization of dentistry has led to a divide between patients and customers. The latter want and expect service, while the former perceive their dental management in the context of a far bigger health picture.

Regrettably implant treatment is often marketed as offering a unique esthetic dimension to achieve best results. This may be misleading, because the role of implant treatment is not a guarantee of an esthetic solution but a useful adjunctive one. In fact, well-planned traditional prosthodontic treatment techniques can be successfully recruited to address the majority of dental esthetic challenges.

The one big convenience that implants offer is the scope offered for ready incorporation of optimal retention and stability into a final treatment plan. Prosthetic teeth can then be placed in desired esthetic locations with minimal concerns for neutral zone directives. This is particularly germane to situations where morphologic and specific biologic changes related to aging, namely advanced residual ridge resorption, circumoral collapse due to altered tissue tone, or neurologic deficits, demand the sort of soft tissue support that would otherwise be unattainable. An obvious example here is the elderly edentulous patient with advanced residual ridge resorption for whom an implant-supported and -retained prosthesis of the fixed or overdenture variety would readily address the attendant esthetic concerns (see chapter 1, Figs 1-1 to 1-3).

Nonetheless, the risk of a fundamental treatment shift to cosmetic commodity status is not entirely without side benefits. For example, the decision to replace missing single or multiple teeth in visible anterior sites (so-called esthetic zones) and where ridge bulk is depleted has already led to the introduction of numerous ingenious surgical reconstructive protocols—both with and without regenerative bone techniques—obviating the need for use of prosthetic materials to simulate missing soft tissues.

# The Oral Ecology

Osseointegration has triggered a new mindset that will significantly change the face of prosthodontic education. The notion of oral ecologic responsibilities, or an "inconvenient truth," is already perceived as paralleling the earth's current and somewhat similar ecologic concerns. This perception is likely to strengthen as the profound differences between a tooth and an implant's attachment mechanism become increasingly self-evident.

The mouth, like the surrounding environment of which it is an integral part, can be regarded as reacting to change with an intervention price that can either enhance or undermine ecologic outcomes. This is no longer an exclusively academic hypothesis; hence clinicians must regard decision making as expanded to include a much broader-based concern with outcomes that are biologically tenable. For example, treatment planning in prosthodontics is based on the consideration of two key questions (Fig 14-2):

1. What is the biomechanical and esthetic price that results from the patient's presenting oral health status?
2. What are the biomechanical risks inherent to the required interventions?

The first question is relatively easy to answer, because any damage encountered by the clinician can be seen and imaged and tested. Disease processes and their sequelae, at their diverse levels of presentation, can be readily studied and the resultant information synthesized into a comprehensive diagnosis. Above all, the resultant intraoral ecologic changes can be reconciled with the patient's systemic health and behavioral considerations. The net result of each such exercise leads to a decision on what an intervention should comprise. The answer to the second question is often more difficult.

Patients are consumers and expect to pay for both correct and ethical guidance and the treatment itself. They often want a say in the treatment plan, and their subjective concerns and wishes as well as their commitment to optimal oral health maintenance must also be viewed in the context of what professionals have to offer. That choice also includes a strong awareness of the inherent biologic price of any prosthodontic intervention. A knee-jerk response to treatment ("Let's replace the missing teeth") is no longer valid in the osseointegration era. The relative ecologic implications of implant-supported prostheses, as compared with tooth- or soft tissue–supported ones, now demands a complex yet more balanced and salutary approach to guiding patients.

The biotechnology that underpins osseointegration and its applications has been successfully harnessed to manage the consequences of dental diseases. Hopefully new biotechnologies will also soon become available to cure caries and periodontal diseases. In the interim, implant preprosthetic surgery and implant prosthodontics are likely to continue to dominate the needs of all those patients who have already lost their teeth or who have remaining dentitions with poor prognoses. Additional concerns still exist, though, regarding the apparent abandon with which implant solutions continue to be promoted.

Recently promoted technologies link computerized tomographic scans to surgical guides and prosthetic delivery, assuring accuracy of implant placement and prosthetic fit within a short time frame; these systems appear to be the ultimate in technologic brilliance and patient convenience. The protocol is likely to prove to be a boon in the hands of experienced specialists, even if the associated price tag may be perceived as excessive. On the other hand, the questions about the repeatability of the approach, the need for such accelerated treatment, and the dangers of its being used by inexperienced dentists suggest cause for much concern. The osseointegration technique has become so attractive that the mantra of "teeth in an

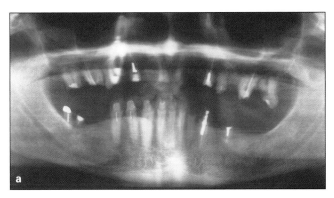
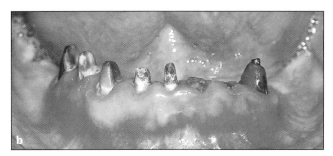

**Fig 14-2** An exploratory panoramic radiograph *(a)* and a mandibular intraoral view *(b)* of a compromised dentition underscore the challenge of reconciling the two factors that confront a clinician who plans a prosthodontic rehabilitation: the consequences of the current oral health status and the biomechanical sequelae of any intervention chosen. Treatment choices range from restoration of the entire dentition to extractions and provision of implant-supported fixed or removable prostheses. The ecologic implications of either treatment will have to be assessed in the context of the patient's oral and systemic health, behavior, economics, age, and overall understanding of the incurred mutual responsibilities for a successful long-term outcome.

hour or a day" runs the risk of distracting the practitioner from the true worth of this biologic breakthrough.

MacEntee[1] recently quoted the French philosopher, Michel Foucault (1926–1984), who wrote that "Medical certainty is based not on the completely observed individuality but on the completely scanned multiplicity of individual facts." Indeed, this ability to scan a multiplicity of individual facts efficiently and reliably is what distinguishes the clinical specialist from the general practitioner. Unfortunately, the profession's collective scanning gaze is imprecise in many areas and at times blind to the wants and needs of the community. It is therefore understandable that a number of responsible clinical educators continue to demand evidence-based approaches that systematically evaluate existing research in the field. For example, it is encouraging to note that simple and easy-to-interpret information about the impact of dental treatment can be acquired from the use of single-item questionnaires. This sort of approach permits quality of evaluation design and outcome measures that are feasible and readily assessed, leading to a hierarchy of core outcome measures that can be universally applied for the benefit of all patients.

## The Research Question

The British statesman Winston Churchill observed that there is nothing wrong with change if it is in the right direction. Change is obviously a constant, but learning is optional. And all of us in the profession can only learn and grow if we em-

brace change that is credible as a result of scientific rigor. In a provocative commentary, "Dancing with the Porcupine: Rules for Governing the University-Industry Relationship,"[2] a distinguished team of authors observes that, while the duty of universities is to seek the truth, the duty of pharmaceutical companies is to make money for their shareholders; the companies that fail to do so go out of business. These authors also assert that universities that subordinate the search for truth to other ends lose credibility and their claim to a privileged place in society. If either institution abandons its fundamental mission, operational imperatives are bound to conflict and failure becomes a risk.

While the commentary addresses the relationship between pharmaceutical companies and universities, its implicit message regarding a health profession's safeguarding of the public interest applies to the dental implant field as well. The authors explicitly sum up their case by stating that:

Research can either serve or subvert public interest. Its findings may advance knowledge and support useful innovation, or be filtered and twisted to support prejudices or gain commercial advantage. The capacities and integrity of researchers, and their universities, can be enhanced or corrupted in the process. Some partnerships are united by an open-minded quest for discovery; others are unholy alliances whereby researchers and universities become handmaidens of industry. Whatever ethical bed we make, we lie in.[2]

There exists today an alarming commercialization of the dental implant field. No other dental technique has been characterized by so much aggressive marketing. This is reflected in the availability of numerous implant systems that lack any form of research track record, particularly long-term treatment outcomes. As a result of the ever-present entrepreneurial spirit and clinical empiricism that abound in the dental profession, implant-supported prostheses threaten to become an automatic response for the management of every form of partial and complete edentulism. Clinical educators and practitioners readily concede that the clinical efficacy of the osseointegration technique is today beyond dispute. However, it must also be recognized that compelling evidence is lacking to support its comprehensive effectiveness with regard to the relative benefits and risks of the various treatment alternatives that are available for patients, third-party providers, and governments.

The profession's most important commodity—intellectual integrity—must be protected by the sorts of commitment or even rules that ensure due diligence. Universities, professional organizations, and scientific journals must continue to be the major sources of clinical education, promoting research involving human subjects that includes definition, disclosure, and management of conflict of interest. This is inarguably the best way to ensure that osseointegration has an ongoing role in redefining so much of the profession's remit.

## Conclusion

The original mandate for writing this book included a partial celebratory agenda. It aimed for a 2007 launch to coincide with the 25th anniversary of the educational introduction of the osseointegration concept. However, efforts to ensure an open-minded analysis and synthesis of intervening developments in the field took a littler longer than hoped for, and the attraction of a quarter century label had to be modified.

Osseointegration was of course born more than 26 years ago, although it is tempting to attribute its unique clinical applications potential to its 1982 Toronto debut. Its subsequent worldwide trajectory ushered in a therapeutic revolution in rehabilitative dentistry. It also ensured exciting and continuing interactions between clinical disciplines and the world of biomaterials.

Per-Ingvar Brånemark's scientific odyssey remains a remarkable example of empirically tested convictions and observa-

tions—a far cry from the currently described, but rarely achieved, standard of randomized controlled clinical trials. Yet he succeeded in changing clinical scientists' and practitioners' traditional convictions about the feasibility and desirability of dental implants. Those of us who were present at the original 1982 symposium will always recall the heady experience of being in the presence of North America's leading academic oral and maxillofacial surgeons and prosthodontists, who came to criticize but stayed to pay tribute.

The objectives of this book were to mine available scientific information and our own collective clinical experiences, to articulate the concerns and convictions that lurk there, and to present them as a coherent package. We also sought to honor the brilliance of one man's scientific ingenuity, personal integrity, and humanism—his journey from the edges of clinical science to the center of both our patients' and our own clinical lives.

## References

1. MacEntee M. Where science fails prosthodontics. Int J Prosthodont 2007; 20:377–381.
2. Lewis S, Baird P, Evans RG, et al. Dancing with the porcupine: Rules for governing the university-industry relationship. CMAJ 2001;165:783–785.

## Recommended Reading

Academy of Osseointegration. State of the Science on Implant Dentistry. [Proceedings of the Consensus Conference on the State of the Science on Implant Dentistry. 3–6 Aug 2006, Oak Brook, IL]. Int J Oral Maxillofac Implants 2007;22(suppl):1–226.

John MT, Reissmann DR, Allen F, Biffar R. The short-term effect of prosthodontic treatment on self-reported oral health status: The use of a single-item questionnaire. Int J Prosthodont 2007;20:507–513.

Nishimura I, Huang Y, Butz F, Ogawa T, Lin A, Wang CJ. Discrete deposition of hydroxyapatite nanoparticles on a titanium implant with predisposing substrate microtopography accelerated osseointegration. Nanotechnology [serial online] 2007;18:245101–245110.

Walton T. Too many cooks and not enough chefs [editorial]. Int J Prosthodont 2007;19:530–531.

Watzek G. Oral implants—Quo vadis? [editorial]. Int J Oral Maxillofac Implants 2006;21:831–832.

Zarb GA, MacEntee M, Anderson JD (eds). On biological and social interfaces in prosthodontics: Proceedings of an international symposium. Int J Prosthodont 2003;16(suppl):1–94.

# APPENDIX

## INTERNET RESOURCES

CHRISTINE WHITE

## EVALUATING WEBSITES

Today, the amount of information found on the Internet increases daily at an exponential rate. How does a health professional locate the most current, authoritative, and relevant material on the Internet? Here are some tips:

- Check the domain in the Internet address to see if the author is commercial, personal, or governmental. For instance, a *.com* address can be either a commercial or personal site (eg, http://www.Google.com). Other Internet address domains include *.edu* (academic institution); *.gov* (US government agency); or *.org* (nonprofit organization).
- Is the website updated regularly? A good website will indicate the date it was last updated.
- Is the information reputable, well-organized, and current? If the site includes other links, are those sources also reliable and well organized? Are any of the links dead?
- What are the credentials of the "author"? Use the same discriminating standards you would apply to print resources such as books or journals. A good website should identify the credentials or authority of the author, whether it is an agency, a company, or an individual.
- What is the purpose of the website: to entertain, to inform, or to persuade?
- What other websites link to this site? One easy method of finding out is to go to http://www.Alexa.com and paste in the Uniform Resource Locator (URL) of the website you are evaluating. Alexa.com will offer statistics on the site, including other websites that link to it, traffic patterns, and page history.
- Does the website provide information about copyright issues and how to obtain permission to reproduce information from the site?

## SEARCHING THE INTERNET EFFICIENTLY

To search the Internet most efficiently, use a good search engine to locate information. Currently, the most popular and largest search engine is Google (http://www.Google.com). The ability of Google to find relevant hits results in part from the search engine's PageRank process, which ranks search results by both the number of webpages linking to it and by the importance of those pages. Google also offers the user an excellent selection of limits to narrow the results of a search.

Here are a few basic suggestions for searching the Internet efficiently using Google:

- To search phrases, such as *dental caries*, use quotation marks (ie, "dental caries"). Google will retrieve results that use the words only as a term or phrase (words positioned next to each other), not as separate words in a text.
- Use the Boolean operator OR (capitalized) to search synonyms (eg, *caries* OR *cavities*). The operator OR can also be used for variations in spelling (eg, *pediatric* OR *paediatric*). The Boolean operator AND is automatic in Google. For instance, if you wish to search two terms, such as *caries* and *fluoride*, type them as *caries fluoride* and Google will interpret the words as *caries* AND *fluoride*. You can also use the Boolean operator NOT to eliminate irrelevant words or phrases (eg, *fluoride* NOT *topical*).
- In Google, you can also limit by language, file format, update frequency, where search terms appear on a webpage, domain, or specific sites (government, military, or university). To utilize these limits, click on *Advanced Search* on the Google home page.

- If you find a relevant hit that is in a foreign language, Google offers a translation feature: On the Google home page, click on *Language Tools*.
- For a copy of Google's "cheat sheet," which offers additional limit features, go to the search engine's home page and search using the term *"cheat sheet" Google*.

# SEARCHING FOR BIOMEDICAL LITERATURE

PubMed (http://www.pubmed.gov) is a database that was developed at the US National Library of Medicine (NLM). Available since 1966, it provides users with access to more than 16 million bibliographic citations for biomedical literature. PubMed is available free to anyone in the world.

PubMed includes Medline, the NLM's biomedical database, which encompasses citations from approximately 5,000 biomedical journals published in the United States and worldwide. Currently, coverage includes citations from 1950 to the present.

PubMed offers users several methods for searching, ranging from easy to difficult. For instance, PubMed can be searched simply by typing in author names, a title, text words, journal titles, or by going to the Medical Subject Headings Database (MeSH Database). If a user has an incomplete citation and wishes to locate the entire reference, the database offers a *Single Citation Matcher* feature. With each citation listed in the results of a search, PubMed includes a *Related Articles* link that automatically lists five article citations that are closely related to the search result.

PubMed also offers a *Limit* tab that has features to narrow search results (eg, language, sex, age, human/animal, date, or publication type); an icon with each hit that identifies whether a citation has an abstract or an electronic link to a free or for-fee full-text article; a *Save Search* function so a search strategy can be rerun at a future date; and an *Auto Alert* feature that allows search strategies to be run automatically daily, weekly, or monthly.

For the novice, tutorials are available on the PubMed home page. An online search manual also can be found on the home page, under the *Help* link. NLM Fact Sheets are also available at http://www.nlm.nih.gov/pubs/factsheets/factsheets.html (alphabetical list) and http://www.nlm.nih.gov/pubs/factsheets/factsubj.html (subject list).

# PROCURING JOURNAL ARTICLES

After you have made a list of articles you want to read, you have several options for finding full-text electronic or paper copies.

## PubMed

The PubMed database offers free full-text articles for selected citations. Free articles are signified by a PubMed icon that is displayed with the search results. To read more about the icon displays, go to http://www.nlm.nih.gov/docline/freehealthlit.html. You can also use PubMed's *Limit* command to restrict your results to free full-text articles.

PubMed provides a *LinkOut* feature in *Abstract* and *Citation* displays of search results. This offers links to online full-text articles from a publisher (usually for a fee). *LinkOut* may also offer a link to an academic library's full-text or paper resources, if the PubMed search is conducted on the academic campus of that library.

The *LinkOut* function will also refer users to free online full-text articles in *PubMed Central* (http://pubmedcentral.gov), a digital archive of biomedical and other science journal literature that has been created by the National Library of Medicine.

A fourth option is *Loansome Doc*, which makes it possible for PubMed users in the United States and abroad to order articles electronically. To initiate the *Loansome Doc* process, contact a library (medical, hospital, or health science) that uses the NLM's *DOCLINE*, which is an automated interlibrary loan request and referral system, to arrange to have article requests routed electronically to yourself. (There may be a fee for each article.) For more information about the *Loansome Doc* process, see http://www.nlm.nih.gov/pubs/factsheets/loansome_doc.html.

## Open-access sites

Users may also find free full-text articles at several open-access websites, which do not require any membership or fee:

- *Biomed Central* (http://www.biomedcentral.com) is an independent publisher that offers free access to peer-reviewed articles published by them as well as to articles published in more than 175 journals.

• *Public Library of Science* (*PLoS:* http://www.plos.org) is a non-profit organization of scientists and physicians that publishes peer-reviewed, open access scientific journals under the following categories: *PLoS Biology*; *PLoS Medicine*; *PLoS Computational Biology*; *PLoS Genetics*; *PLoS Pathogens*, *PLoS Neglected Tropical Diseases*; *PLoS Clinical Trials*; and *PLoS ONE* (reports of primary research from all scientific and medical disciplines).

• *Highwire Press* (http://highwire.stanford.edu) is currently the largest repository, with more than 1,000 peer-reviewed journals and 4.3 million free full-text articles. Highwire Press is a division of Stanford University Libraries.

• *Directory of Open Access Journals* (*DOAJ:* http://www.doaj.org) is a service that offers more than 2,700 journals in its directory with access to more than 134,487 full-text articles.

• *Journal Storage* (*JSTOR:* http://www.jstor.org) is a free archive of back issues of several hundred academic journals whose articles have been digitized. JSTOR's collection does not usually include current or recently published articles; there is typically a 1- to 5-year gap.

• *Scientific Electronic Library Online* (*SciELO:* http://www.scielo.org) offers free access to articles from selected journals published in Brazil, Spain, Cuba, and Chile.

• *Japan Science and Technology Information Aggregator, Electronic* (*J-STAGE:* http://www.jstage.go.jp/browse) includes full-text electronic journals as well as reports and proceedings from some of Japan's scientific societies.

• *British Medical Journal Online* (http://journals.bmj.com/subscriptions/countries.shtml) offers low- and middle-income countries free access to full-text journals published by BMJ Publishing Group Limited. See the website for a list of the countries whose institutions are eligible for free access.

• *Health InterNetwork Access to Research Initiative* (*HINARI:* http://www.who.int/hinari/en/). This website was created by the World Health Organization and major publishers to facilitate the full-text access of more than 3,700 biomedical and health literature journals.

• *Popline, Information & Knowledge for Optimal Health* (*INFO*) *Project, Johns Hopkins Center for Communication Programs* (http://db.jhuccp.org/popinform/aboutpl.html) offers developing countries free access to full-text articles. Topics include reproductive health, population and demographic issues,

human immunodeficiency virus (HIV) and acquired immunodeficiency syndrome (AIDS), and environmental health.

• *FreeMedicalJournals.com* (http://www.freemedicaljournals.com) enables users to view free online full-text journals and search for journals by title, language, or specialty.

## Document delivery suppliers

There are numerous document delivery suppliers who can provide articles worldwide for a fee. To find the websites for other national libraries that may offer document delivery services, go to http://www.ifla.org/II/natlib.htm for a list produced by the International Federation of Library Associations and Institutions. Alternatively, try a Google search using the search phrase *"national libraries"*. This will produce hits with lists of national libraries worldwide and their websites, if available.

To find additional document suppliers, try a Google search using the search phrase *"document delivery suppliers"*. The following is a list of some suppliers:

• *National Library of Medicine* (*Loansome Doc*). See the explanation in the section on PubMed.

• *British Library Direct* (http://direct.bl.uk/bld/Home.do) has full-text data from 20,000 of the most popular journal titles at the British Library. If an article is available in an electronic format, it can be purchased by credit card and downloaded immediately. Paper copies of articles will take longer to receive because they must be scanned.

• *Canada Institute for Scientific and Technical Information* (*CISTI:* http://cisti-icist.nrc-cnrc.gc.ca/main_e.html) offers document delivery for all areas of science, technology, engineering, and medicine. Payment may be made by credit card or monthly billing.

• *BioDox Document Delivery Services* (http://www.biodox.com/) provides delivery of articles related to biologic, chemical, and pharmaceutical sciences.

• *ISI Document Solution* (http://scientific.thomson.com/products/ds/) offers several methods of delivery (electronic, mail, fax, or courier).

# INDEX